HISTOLOGY LAB ATLAS

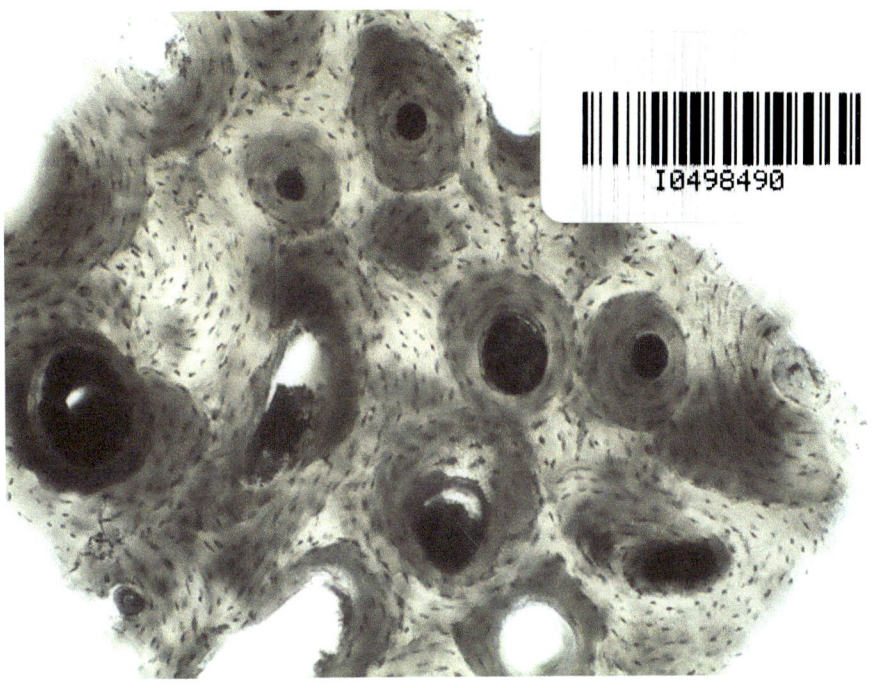

By

MICHAEL HARRELL, M.S.

© Professor Michael T Harrell, all rights reserved.

No part of this book may be reproduced, stored, or transmitted by any means without the written permission of the author.

Published December 2012

Dedication

To my wife for her love, dedication, and support.

TABLE OF CONTENTS

INTRODUCTION TO TISSUES	8
ADIPOSE TISSUE (connective tissue)	16-19
ADRENAL GLAND (capsule, cortex, medulla)	20-22
ALVEOLI (simple squamous epithelial)	23
APPENDIX (smooth muscle and mucosa)	24-25
ARTERY (elastic tissue)	26-27
BLADDER (transitional epithelial tissue)	28-30
BLOOD (connective tissue)	31-36
BONE MARROW (connective tissue)	37-38
CANCELLOUS BONE (also P. 157) (connective tissue)	39
CARDIAC MUSCLE (intercalated disks, nuclei)	40-43
CEREBELLUM (nervous tissue)	44-47
CEREBRUM (nervous tissue)	48-50
CERVIX (stratified squamous and smooth muscle)	51-52
CHROMOSOMES	53-54
CILIATED PSEUDOSTRATIFIED (epithelial tissue)	55-57
COCHLEA (Scala vestibule, scala tympani, bone)	58
COLON (mucosa, submucosa, smooth muscle)	59-61
COMPACT BONE (connective tissue)	62-64

DIAPHRAGM MUSCLE (skeletal muscle)	65
ELASTIC TISSUE (elastic fibers)	66-67
ELASTIC CARTILAGE (chondrocytes, elastic fibers)	68-69
EPIDIDYMIS (epithelial cells)	70-71
ESOPHAGUS (stratified squamous, submucosa)	72-74
ESOPHAGEAL CARDIAC JUNCTION (strat. sq.)	75-76
FALLOPIAN TUBES (ISTHMUS) (simple columnar)	77-79
GALLBLADDER (simple columnar, lumen)	80
GOBLET CELLS (goblet cells, lamina propria)	81-82
HYPOPHYSIS (PITUITARY GLAND) (more P. 127)	83-84
INTESTINE (simple columnar, smooth muscle)	85-87
KIDNEYS (simple cuboidal, lumen)	88-89
LARGE INTESTINE (simple columnar, glands)	90-92
LIVER (central vein, hepatic cords, sinusoids)	93-96
LOOSE CONNECTIVE TISSUE (collagen, fibroblasts)	97-99
LUNG (alveoli, simple squamous, carbon)	100-102
LUNG WITH CARBON (smokers lung)	103-104
LYMPH NODE (capsule, cortex, medulla, lymphocytes)	105-107
MAMMARY GLANDS (stratified columnar epithelial)	108
MITOSIS (all stages)	109-114

MOTOR END PLATES   (striations, axons)   115-116

NERVE   (axons)   117-118

OVARY – MATURE FOLLICLE   (oocyte, antrum)   119-120

PANCREAS   (pancreatic islets)   121-124

PARATHYROID GLAND   (thyroid, parathyroid)   125-126

PITUITARY GLAND (ANTERIOR)   (more P. 83)   127

PROSTATE GLAND   (smooth muscle, epithelial tissue)   128-129

RECTUM   (simple columnar, goblet cells, glands)   130-131

SCALP   (epidermis, dermis, hypodermis, strata)   132-134

SIMPLE COLUMNAR EPITHELIAL   (goblet cells)   135-136

SKELETAL MUSCLE   (striations, nuclei)   137-140

SKIN   (epidermis, dermis, strata)   141-142

SMOOTH MUSCLE   (nuclei)   143-145

SPINAL CORD   (white matter, grey matter, neurons)   146-152

SPINAL NERVE   (axons)   153-154

SPLEEN   (red & white pulp, capsule, trabeculae)   155-156

SPONGY BONE – CANCELLOUS BONE   (trabeculae)   157

STOMACH   (simple columnar, gastric pits, tunics)   158-162

SUBMANDIBULAR GLANDS   (simple cuboidal)   163

SWEAT GLANDS   (simple cuboidal cells)   164-165

TENDON (dense regular collagenous connective)	166
TESTIS (seminiferous tubules, Leydig cells)	167-170
THREADS (3 colors at different depths)	171
THYMUS GLAND (cortex, medulla, trabeculae)	172-174
THYROID GLAND (thyroid follicles, parafollicular cells)	175-176
TONGUE (stratified squamous, taste buds)	177-178
TONSILS (lymphocytes)	179-180
TRACHEA (Ciliated pseudostratified layer)	181
URETER (Transitional epithelium, lamina propria)	182-183
VAGINA (stratified squamous, lamina propria)	184-185
VENA CAVA (tunica intima, media, adventitia)	186

There are many tissue types in the human body, and we want to discuss the primary tissues.

The tissues in our body can be grouped into 4 different categories: epithelial, connective, muscular and nervous. Every tissue of the body can be placed into one of these four categories. Make sure you can place any tissue into one of those four tissue types. Slides often contain several tissues, so don't let that confuse you.

1. EPITHELIAL TISSUE
Epithelial tissue will be found in many places of the body. Primarily you will find it covering and lining most surfaces of the body. Skin will come to mind first and that is a great example of epithelial tissue. Remember this tissue is found in many places. If you look at the four body systems which open to the outside of the body (respiratory, digestive, urinary, and reproductive) they all have passageways opening to the outside of the body. All of these passageways are lined with epithelial tissues. Also, most glands of the body are made of epithelial tissue.

Even though this tissue is creating a barrier in many places, don't think that they don't allow for the passage of materials. In some places, like the skin, the cells allow very little to pass through them. In many other places they do allow for passage. Thick layers will always prevent the passage of materials, where thin layers will allow for passage.

Epithelial tissue always has certain characteristics. Make sure you are familiar with the characteristics of each of the tissues. In epithelial tissues you will see the following:
- Very little space between the cells. Epithelial cells are tightly packed, so they can make good barriers. Some of these binding connections are desmosomes, hemidesmosomes, gap junctions and tight junctions. Other tissues are not as tightly packed as epithelial tissues are.
- Most epithelial tissues will have a structure called the basement membrane. This is a thin layer which will bind it to another tissue and guides it during cellular repair. Not all epithelial tissues have it, but it is a characteristic of most. A basement membrane won't be found with any other tissue type.

- Blood vessels don't penetrate epithelial tissues. Why is this? Many epithelial tissues are superficial and on the surface of something. Since they are superficial, you don't want blood vessels penetrating them. If blood vessels did, it would be easy to lose blood and get infections into them.
- Epithelial tissues have many proteins binding them together. With all of these binding structures, it holds them together tightly, making a good barrier.
-Because these cells are covering and protecting structures, the cells are always being lost on their surface. Because of this, the cells are almost always in mitosis.

A few terms will describe most epithelial tissues and you need to know what the terms mean. There are three terms which describe epithelial cell layers and three which describe cell shapes.

The three terms describing cell layers are:
Simple – 1 layer
Stratified – 2 or more layers
Pseudostratified – 1 layer. The term means falsely stratified because it looks like two layers. This type will often have cilia on the surface and mucous is often what the cilia are moving. They will often have goblet cells with them. Goblet cells do one thing, make mucous.

The three terms describing cell shapes are:
Squamous – means flat
Cuboidal – cube shape
Columnar – tall and thin, like a column in front of a house
In the description of most epithelial tissues, you will find one word from the first group and one word from the second group. Examples would include:
Simple squamous epithelial tissue = one layer of flat cells
Simple columnar = one layer of column shaped cells
Stratified squamous = many layers of flat cells
Make sure you understand the meaning of these six terms. You will without a doubt, have questions concerning the meaning of each.

Another type of epithelial tissue, which the above terms don't describe are transitional epithelial tissue. This special type of epithelial tissue is capable of changing its number of cell layers and cell shape. That is why it's called transitional. If something is going through a transition, it is changing. This special tissue is found in the urinary system and allows for expansion. Your urinary bladder has to be able to expand if it is to fill with urine.

   Where you find epithelial tissues making glands, you will find them in two types.
Endocrine glands – glands found within the body producing hormones. These glands will be discussed in detail when you get to the endocrine system. These glands release their products into the spaces surrounding the cells and enter the blood.

   Exocrine glands – glands with a duct leading to the surface of something. Many of these glands are found in the skin. Examples would be sweat glands, sebaceous (oil) glands, mammary glands and ceruminous (ear) glands.
   Exocrine glands come in three forms:
-Merocrine – glands which use exocytosis (vesicles) to secrete materials. Ex-sweat glands
-Apocrine – glands which pinch off a piece of their cell with the materials in them. Ex-mammary glands
-Holocrine – glands were the entire cell falls away into the duct. Ex-sebaceous glands
Make sure you know how the materials are released and an example of each.

2. CONNECTIVE TISSUE

   Connective tissue is the most varied tissue in function and number of locations. There are more tissues within this category than any of the others by far. If you are ever asked to place a tissue into a category and you don't know where it goes, then put it in this one. Connective tissues can often be found connecting other tissues together, thus the name. For example, tendons connect bones to muscles, ligaments connect bone to bone, blood connects most tissues of the body, etc. Many other functions can be performed by this tissue.

Inside the connective tissues you will find an abundance of extracellular matrix. This means that there is much more space between the cells. This is the opposite of epithelial tissue, which has little extracellular space.

The cell names of connective tissues have some terms within them, you need to be familiar with. In connective tissue cell names, you will find the suffixes: blasts, clasts and cytes. Any cell name with blast in it will be a building cell, any with clast in its name will be a breaking down cell and any cyte cell will maintain a tissue. For example, in bones you will find three big cell types: osteoblasts, osteoclasts and osteocytes. Osteoblasts build bone, osteoclasts break down bone and osteocytes maintain bone (meaning the build small amounts). Don't forget those suffixes, they can serve you well in determining cell physiology.

Along with the cells of connective tissues, you will also find several common fibers.
- Collagen is the most common connective tissue fiber and the most abundant protein in the body. Collagen gives strength to tissues. Think of them as steel cables. A steel cable will bend but it won't stretch, this is where the strength comes from.

-Elastin (elastic) fibers are a common fiber which is very flexible. Think of elastin fibers as rubber bands. These fibers will stretch and give flexibility to things such as your arteries.

-Reticular fibers are a type of fine collagen, found mostly in the lymphatic system.

Connective tissues found in the body include the following:
- Adipose tissue – this is what we commonly call fat tissue. Adipocytes are the fat cells you find in adipose tissue. We have adipose tissue to store energy, insulate the body (hold in heat) and make a cushion around deeper structures. In the first few years of our lives, we have a special type of adipose tissue called brown adipose tissue. It is specialized to produce heat in the body.

- Bone tissue – Bone is the hardest, densest tissue in the body. Because it is so hard it is often found protecting deeper structures. Bone comes in two types: compact and cancellous.
Compact bone is a type of bone where the tissue is very compact, with no spaces within it. When you see a histology slide of this bone, it is the one that looks like tree stumps. You will find compact surrounding all bones.

Bone is composed mostly of two materials: collagen (1/3) and hydroxyapatite (2/3). The collagen gives our bones flexibility, and the hydroxyapatite makes it hard.
Cancellous bone is also called spongy bone because it looks a bit like a sponge. Think about all the spaces found within a sponge, which is what this bone looks like.

- Reticular tissue is a tissue full of reticular fibers. If you want to find this tissue, look to the lymphatic system, and bone marrow.

- Loose connective tissue - also called areolar tissue. This tissue gets its name because the fibers have lots of space in between them. Look at any picture of loose connective tissue and you will see all the space between the fibers.

-Dense connective tissue – This tissue gets its name because the fibers are tightly packed together. This tissue is the opposite of the loose tissue. Dense tissue can be found as regular or irregular. Regular dense connective tissue is where most of the fibers are oriented in the same direction, like in a tendon or ligament. Irregular dense connective tissue is where most of the fibers are oriented in many directions.

-Elastic tissue – where the tissue is filled with elastic fibers. This tissue will stretch very well. Arteries have large amounts of elastic tissue in them. Our vocal cords have dense regular elastic tissue.
- Blood – The only tissue in the body that flows like a fluid because it has so much water in its matrix. Blood connects almost all tissues of the body. Blood is composed of plasma (the watery part of the blood) and the formed elements (the cells of the blood). Blood cells will consist of red blood cells, white blood cells and platelets.

- Hemopoietic tissue – This tissue is what we commonly call bone marrow. This is where all of the blood cells are made. There are two types of bone marrow in the body. When we are young, we have red bone marrow, but as we pass maturity, we have more yellow bone marrow. They are the same tissue, but yellow marrow has more adipose tissue in it and red has less adipose tissue.

- Cartilage – This is a strong tissue composed of cells called chondrocytes. Cartilage doesn't contain blood vessels or nerves. Since this tissue is often found in pressure points, it would be useless to put blood vessels and nerves in them. Three types of cartilage are found in the body.
  Hyaline cartilage – This is the second strongest tissue in the body, just after bone. In between bones where they meet, and the embryo skeleton are common sites for this tissue.
  Elastic cartilage – A type of tissue which contains large amounts of elastic fibers. The ears and nose have large amounts of this tissue. That is why those body parts are so flexible.
  Fibrocartilage – Cartilage found in joints under high compression. The disks in between the bodies of our vertebrae are good examples of this tissue. This tissue forms cushions in some joints, acting as shock absorbers. If you ever felt something pop in your knee or jaw, that was fibrocartilage.

3. MUSCLE
  Muscle comes in three forms in the body.
Skeletal – This is the most abundant of the 3 muscle types and is always attached to bone. Skeletal muscle makes about 40% of our total body weight. It has more than one nucleus (peripherally located), had bold stripes on it (striations), is under voluntary control and has a round shape like a pipe. This muscle is what we move our body parts with.

Cardiac – This muscle is only found in the heart. In the heart it's generating pressure to move our blood. These cells have one nucleus, are centrally located and are round in shape. This muscle is involuntary, meaning you can't control it with your conscious thought.

Smooth muscle – This muscle is found in more locations than any other muscle type. Because it is found in so many places, its functions are varied. Much of it is in our digestive system, that is what moves materials through our GI tract. This muscle has a spindle shape to the cells. It has one nucleus per cell and is also involuntary.

4. NERVOUS TISSUE

The nervous system contains many cells, but the most important ones are the neurons. These are what you may call brain cells, but they are found in many places other than the brain. A neuron has 3 main parts to it. These parts are the cell body (soma), dendrite (where neurons receive signals) and the axon (the output part of the neuron).

In addition to the neurons, you will find a group of cells called glial or neuroglial cells. These are any cell in the nervous system that isn't a neuron. They are varied and have many functions. When we get to the nervous system, we will go over them.

Neurons are also classified in different ways. One classification is based on the structure of the cell. Some neurons have many dendrites (multipolar cells), some have one dendrite (bipolar cells) and some have no dendrites (unipolar cells). The number of dendrites is all that varies in this structural classification. The bipolar and unipolar are easily confused. Bipolar get their name because they have two poles, one input (1 dendrite) and one output (1 axon). Unipolar only have an axon, thus unipolar.

Epithelial tissues of the body form membranes in many areas and you need to know them.
1. Serous membranes – These are the same membranes discussed earlier in chapter 2. The membranes which surround organs and are found in enclosed body cavities. The pericardial, pleural and

peritoneal cavities have these visceral (inner) and parietal (outer) membranes. The membranes and fluid reduce friction and hold the organs in place.

2. Mucous membranes – These are the membranes lining the body systems, which have openings to the outside of the body. The linings of the respiratory, digestive, urinary, and reproductive systems all have these membranes.

3. Synovial membranes – These membranes will be found in some of the joints of the body. The membrane will release a fluid containing hyaluronic acid. This acid makes the cartilage in the joints very slippery, and this will reduce friction.

Inflammation
When a tissue is damaged for any reason, it will become inflamed. Inflammation is caused by materials moving from the cardiovascular system into the tissue. When tissues are damaged, chemicals of inflammation are released. These chemicals work to make blood vessels dilate (bringing more blood into a tissue) and make the vessels more permeable (allowing more to move out of the blood). You want more blood in a damaged tissue for the following reasons:
1. Bringing in more red blood cells, delivers more oxygen to cells, which will be needed for repair.
2. Bringing in more white blood cells, will allow for more dead cells and foreign invaders to be destroyed.
3. Bringing in more platelets will help to stop blood loss.
4. Bringing in more plasma will bring in many materials.

The signs of inflammation are redness, heat, pain, swelling and disturbance of function.

ADIPOSE TISSUE

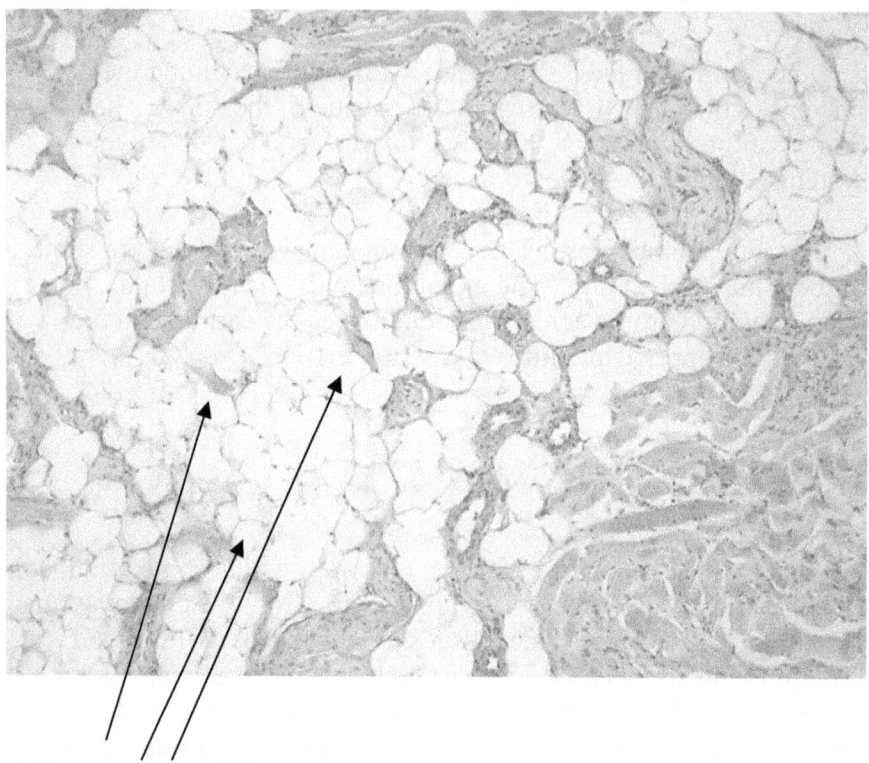

Adipocyte (fat cells)

Adipose tissue is a type of connective tissue.

Adipocytes shown at 100X

Notice the empty appearance of the adipose cells.

Adipose tissue is easy to distinguish from other tissues. The hollow appearance is unique to this tissue.

Adipose tissue has many functions; one of these functions is to cover internal organs acting as a shock absorber for sudden blows to the body.

ADIPOSE TISSUE

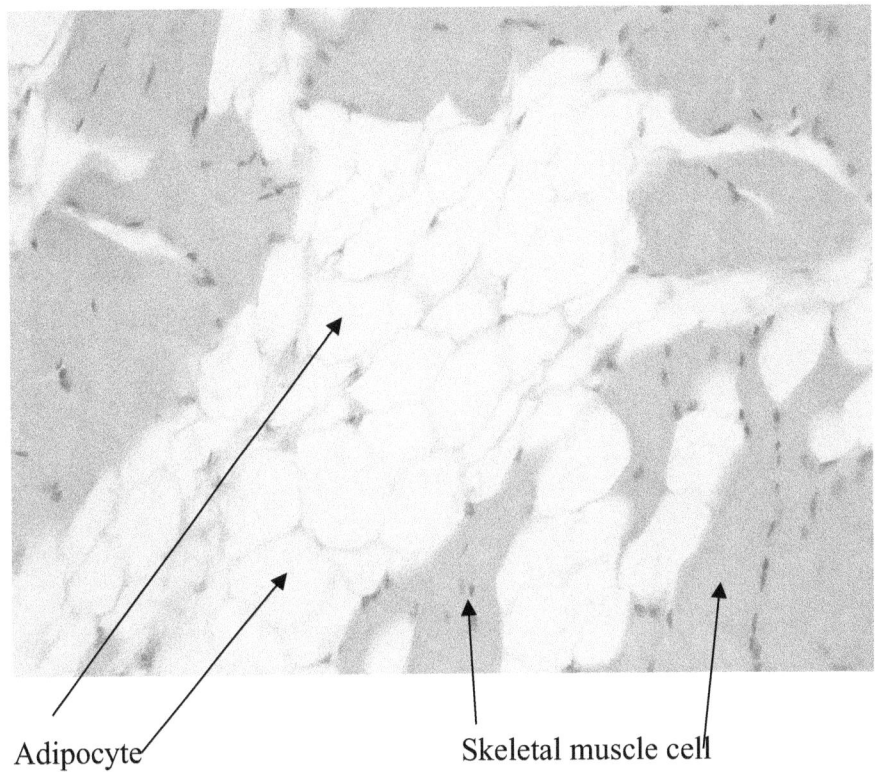

Adipocyte   Skeletal muscle cell

Adipose tissue is a type of connective tissue.

Shown at 400X

Adipose tissue is composed of cells called adipocytes.

Adipocytes are fat cells.

This picture contains adipocytes and skeletal muscle cells.

The skeletal muscle cells are seen in cross section, which is why they may look odd. We are looking into the ends of the skeletal muscle cells.

ADIPOSE TISSUE

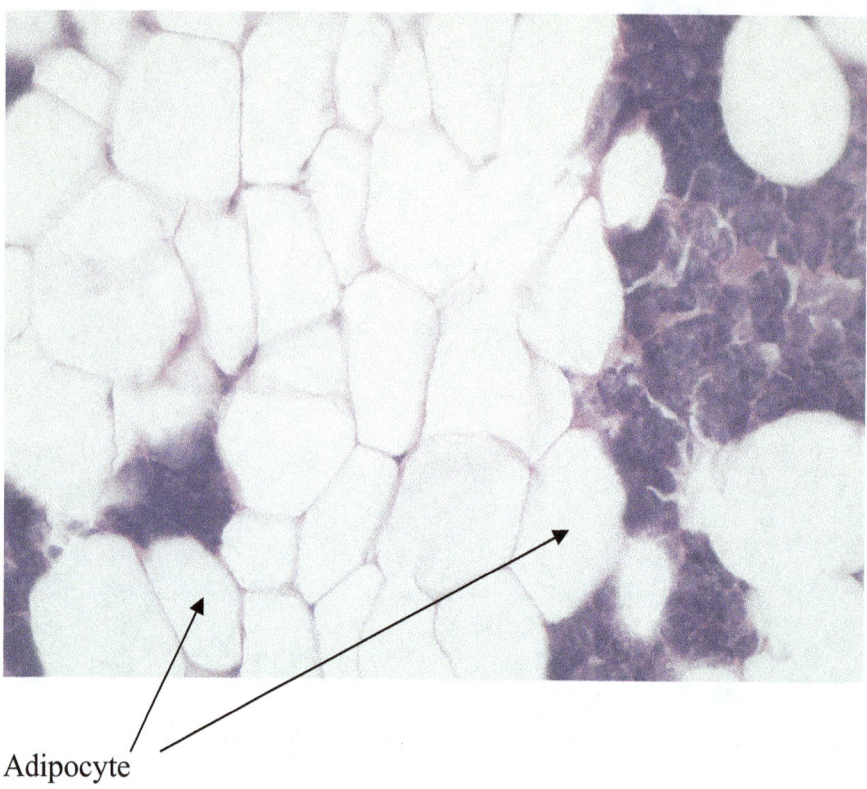

Adipocyte

Adipose tissue is a type of connective tissue.

Adipose tissue at 400X

Notice how the adipocytes look like empty cells.

They have an empty appearance and look like empty cells, but of course they are filled with fats (adipose tissue).

The adipose tissue often looks like a honeycomb.

ADIPOSE TISSUE

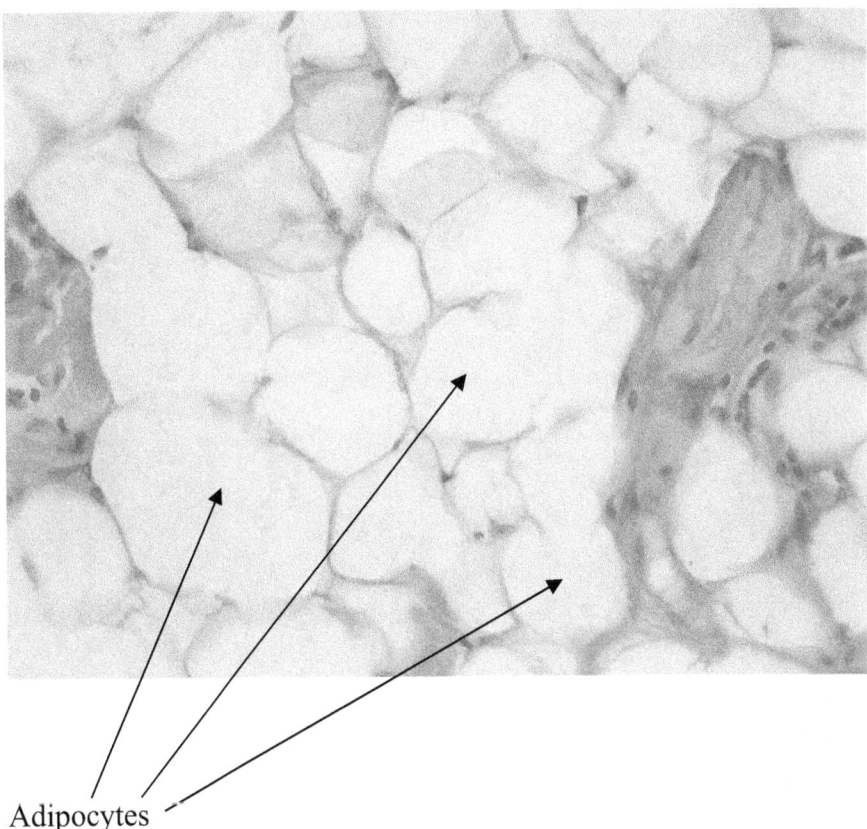

Adipocytes

Adipose tissue at 400X

Adipose tissue is also known as fat tissue. This tissue is filled with fat cells called adipocytes.

Adipocytes store energy, provide a cushion deep to the skin and insulate the body to hold in heat.

Much of our adipose tissue is found just deep to the skin. Here it acts to insulate and cushion the deeper structures.

ADRENAL GLAND

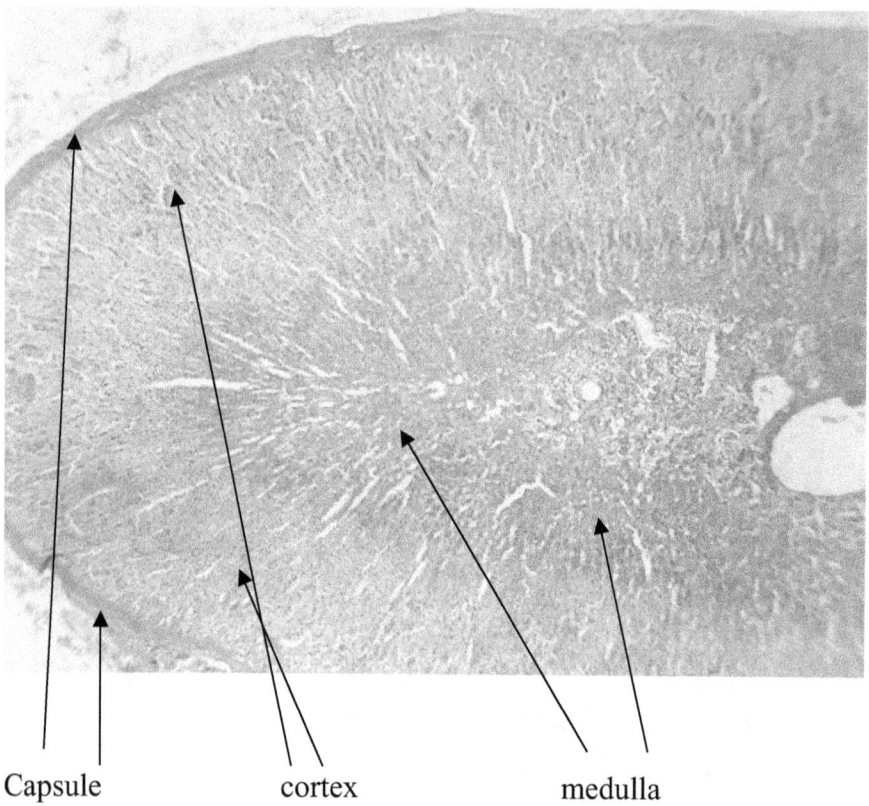

Capsule   cortex   medulla

Adrenal gland 40X

The adrenal glands rest on the superior poles of the kidneys.

The adrenal glands consist of an adrenal cortex and adrenal medulla.

The adrenal cortex releases cortisol, aldosterone, and androgens.

The adrenal medulla releases epinephrine and norepinephrine. It is also part of the sympathetic nervous system.

ADRENAL GLAND

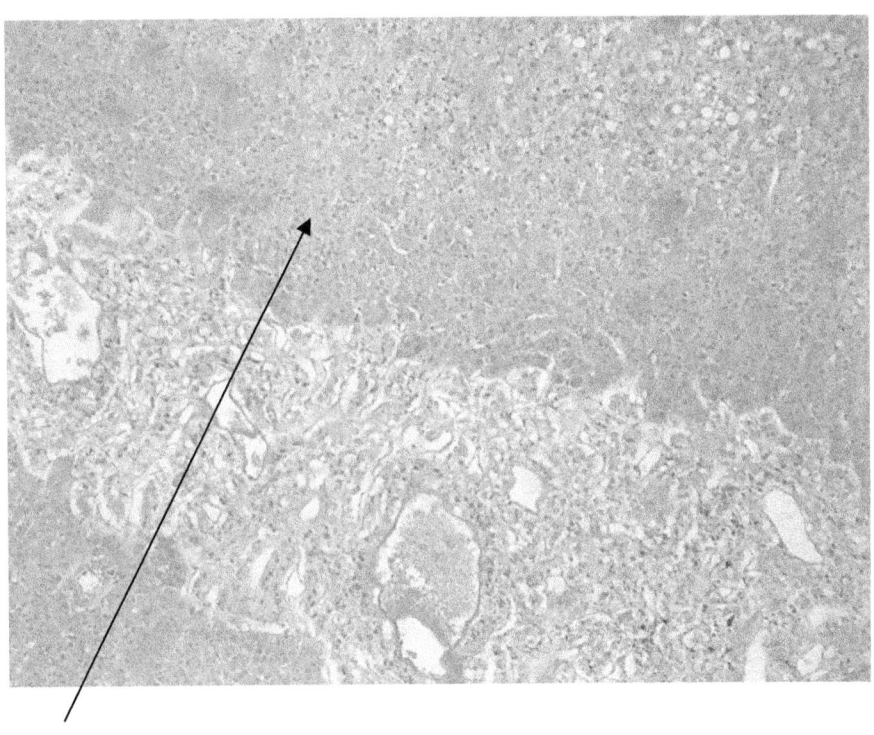

medulla

Adrenal gland at 100X

Adrenal medulla magnified from previous slide.

The adrenal cortex releases cortisol, aldosterone, and androgens.

The adrenal medulla releases epinephrine and norepinephrine.

ADRENAL GLAND

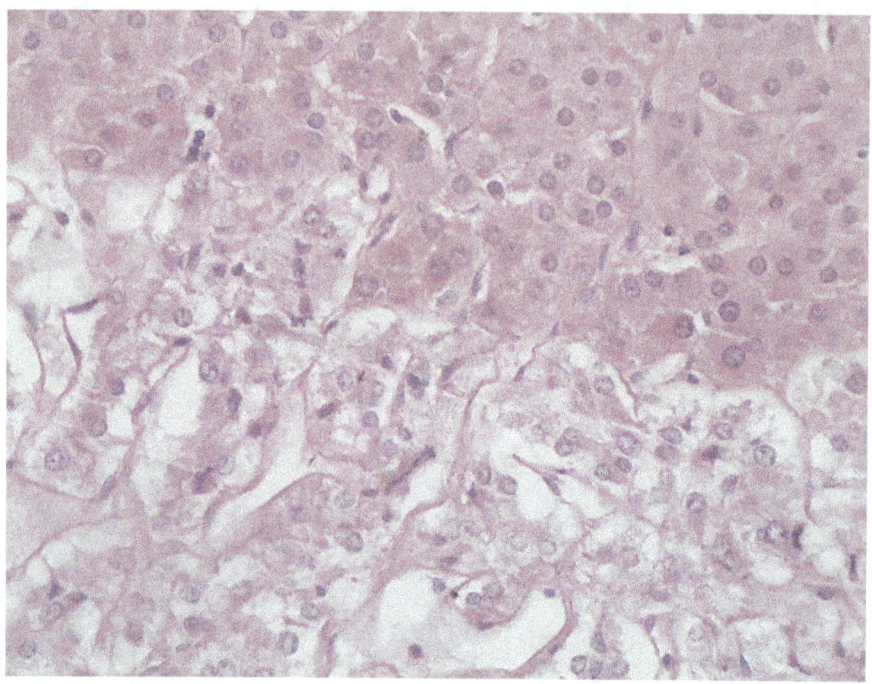

Adrenal gland at 400X

Adrenal medulla magnified from previous slide.

The adrenal cortex releases cortisol, aldosterone and androgens.

The adrenal medulla releases epinephrine and norepinephrine.

ALVEOLI

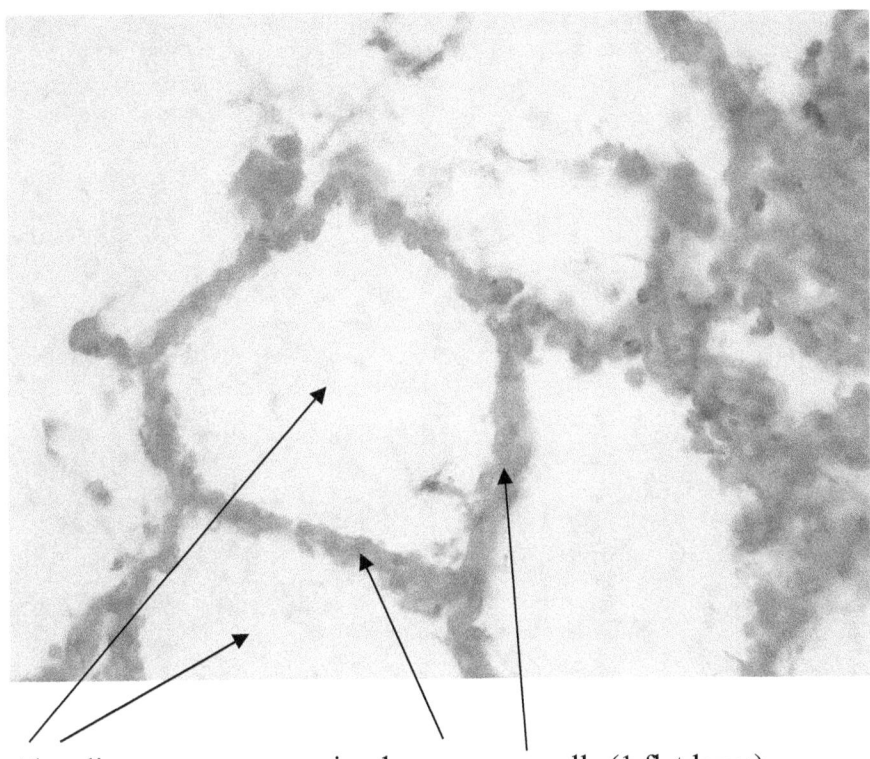

Alveoli   simple squamous cells (1 flat layer)

See lungs for more pictures of simple squamous tissue. This is an epithelial tissue type.

Alveoli at 400X. The alveoli are the tiny air sacs within the lungs.

The alveoli are where oxygen, carbon dioxide and other materials will swap between the air we breathe in and the blood in the pulmonary capillaries.

The walls of the alveoli are made mostly of simple squamous epithelial cells. Remember that simple layers are 1 cell in thickness and squamous cells are flat. This one flat layer of cells is a very thin barrier, and the body puts very thin barriers where it wants materials to move.

APPENDIX

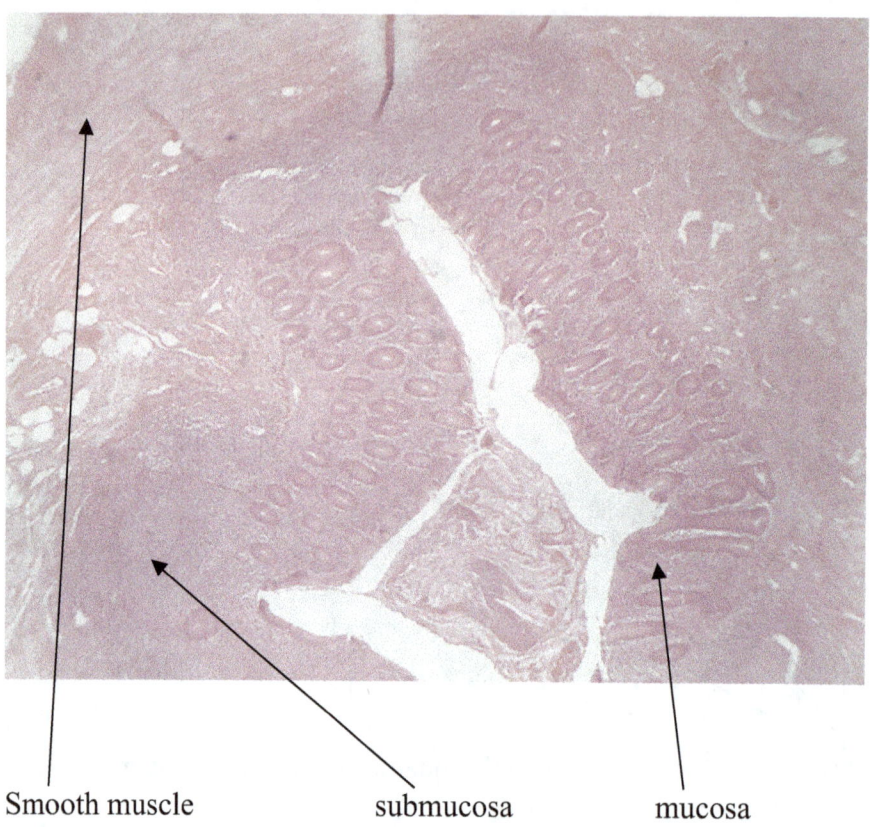

Smooth muscle   submucosa   mucosa

Appendix at 40X

The function of the appendix is debated among physiologists. Some believe the structure is vestigial and nonfunctional. Others believe it acts as a reservoir for helpful bacteria. Other theories exist also.

APPENDIX

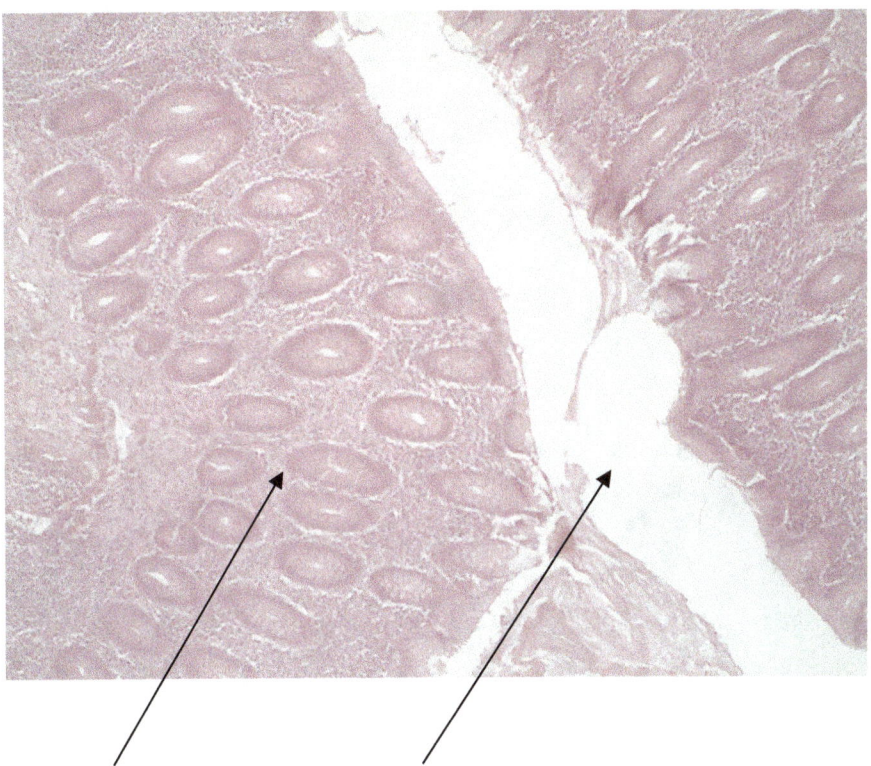

Mucosa layer   lumen (hollow inside)

Magnified view of the mucosa region.

Appendix at 100X

The appendix is attached to the cecum, which is the first part of the large intestine.

The function of the appendix is debated among physiologists. Some believe the structure is vestigial and nonfunctional. Others believe it acts as a reservoir for helpful bacteria. Other theories exist also.

ARTERY

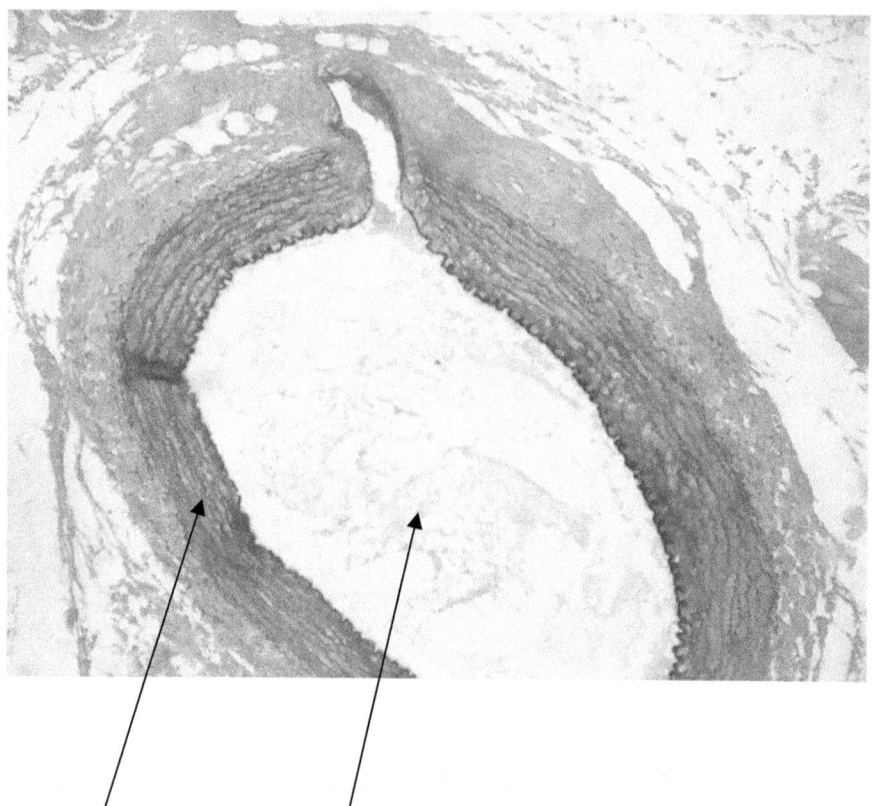

Artery at 100X   Lumen (inside) of the artery.

Notice the thick walls of the artery. An artery wall is much thicker than the wall of a vein. Most of the wall is smooth muscle.

Notice the wrinkled appearance on the inside of the artery. This wrinkled appearance shows how the inner wall allowed for expansion, when blood was applying pressure to the inner walls.

The dark appearance of the artery wall is due to the presence of elastic fibers. Arteries are very elastic, so they can handle the pressure of the blood within.

The lumen is where the blood was flowing.

ARTERY

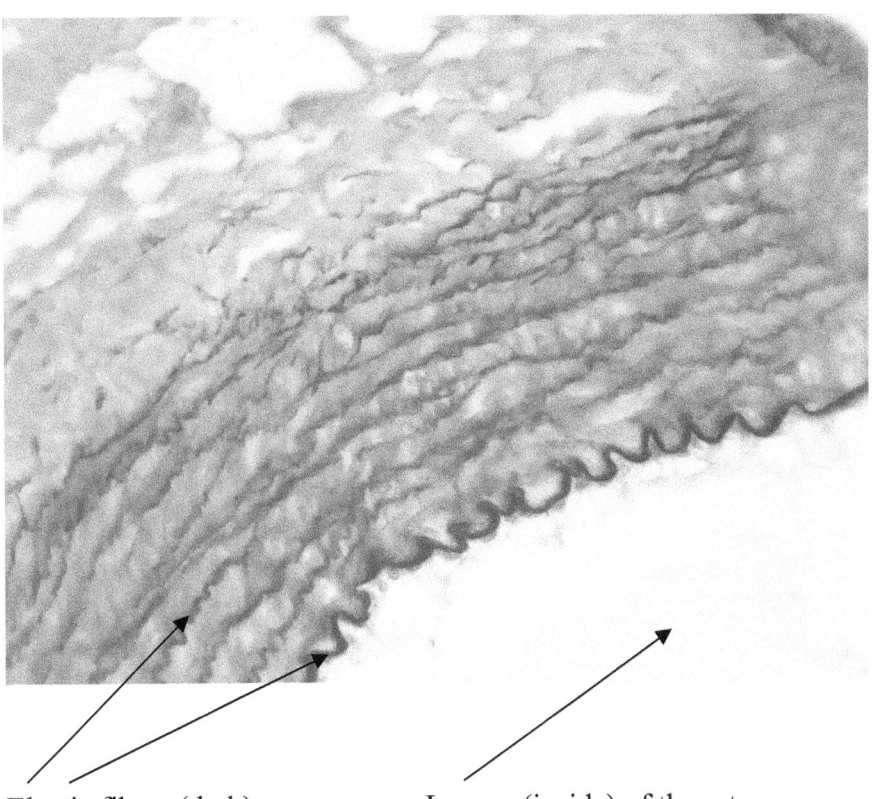

Elastic fibers (dark)   Lumen (inside) of the artery.

Artery at 400X

Arteries are blood vessels which take blood away from the heart. Veins are blood vessels which return blood back to the heart.

Arteries come in three major types: elastic, muscular and arterioles. The large elastic arteries are found close to the heart and are under the greatest amount of pressure. The medium muscular arteries are where much of the vasodilation and vasoconstriction takes place to alter blood flow to organs. The arterioles are the smallest of arteries and the last artery before a capillary.

BLADDER

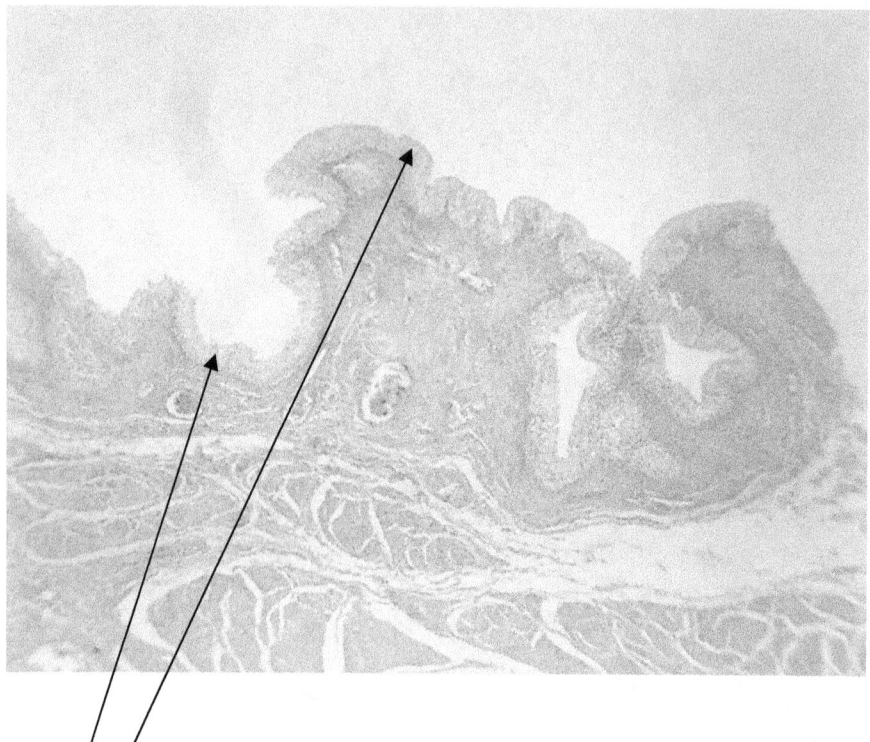

Transitional epithelial layer (layer changes)

Urinary bladder at 40X (bladder is empty)

Notice the layer of transitional epithelial tissue. Transitional epithelial tissue can change in number of cell layers and cell shape. When the bladder is empty the layer is stratified cuboidal. When the bladder fills the cells unfold and change to a few squamous cell layers.

Transitional epithelial tissue is found in the urinary system, where room for expansion is needed.

The urinary bladder is mostly smooth muscle.

BLADDER

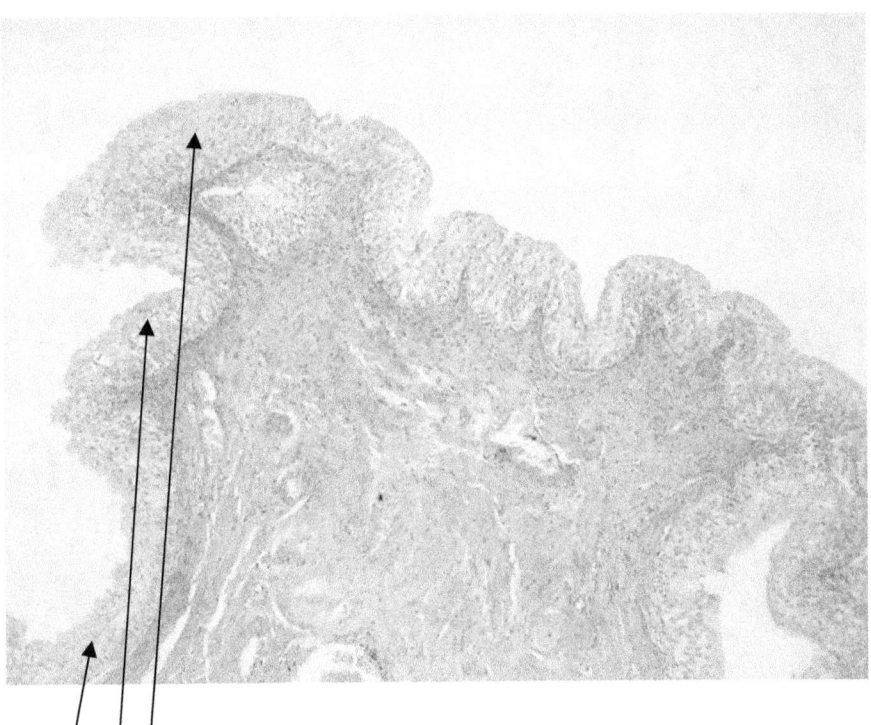

Transitional epithelial tissue (layer changes)

Urinary bladder at 100X (bladder is empty)

The urinary bladder is made mostly of a smooth muscle called the detrusor muscle. The smooth muscle like others is under involuntary control when we are born, but we learn how to control it voluntarily as we grow. Early in life the detrusor muscle will contract automatically, and this autonomic response is called the micturition reflex.

The inferior surface of the bladder has a triangular shaped region called the trigone. The trigone is a triangular shaped region formed by the entrance of the two ureters and the exit point for the urethra.

BLADDER

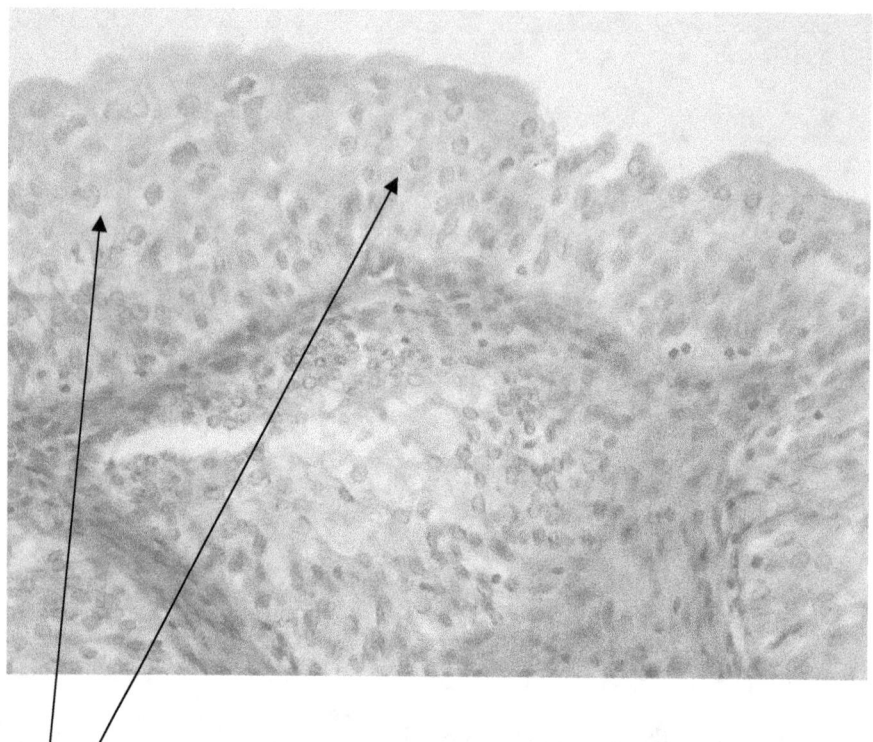

Transitional epithelial tissue (layer changes)

Urinary bladder at 400X (bladder is empty)

As the urinary bladder fills with urine the transitional epithelium will unfold and this allows room for expansion.

BLOOD

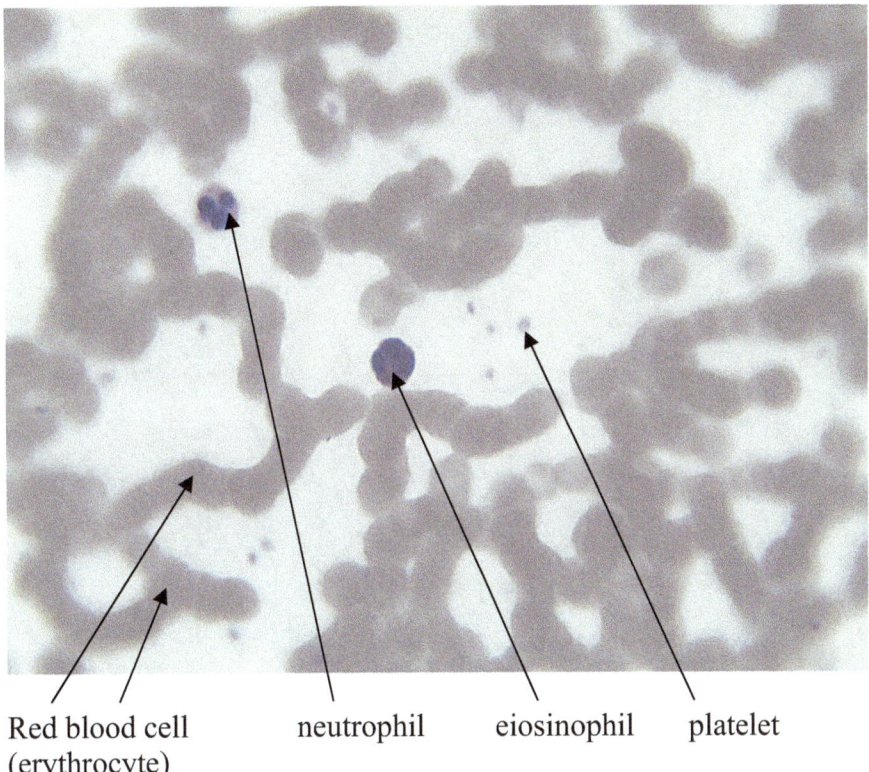

Red blood cell   neutrophil   eiosinophil   platelet
(erythrocyte)

Blood at 1000X

Blood is a connective tissue and makes about 8% of our body weight.

Neutrophils are identified by the 3-5 lobes in the nucleus.

Eiosinophils are identified by the 2 identical lobes and being very grainy.

Platelets are just tiny fragments of cells.

White blood cells come in 5 major groups: neutrophils, eosinophils, basophils, lymphocytes, monocytes.

BLOOD

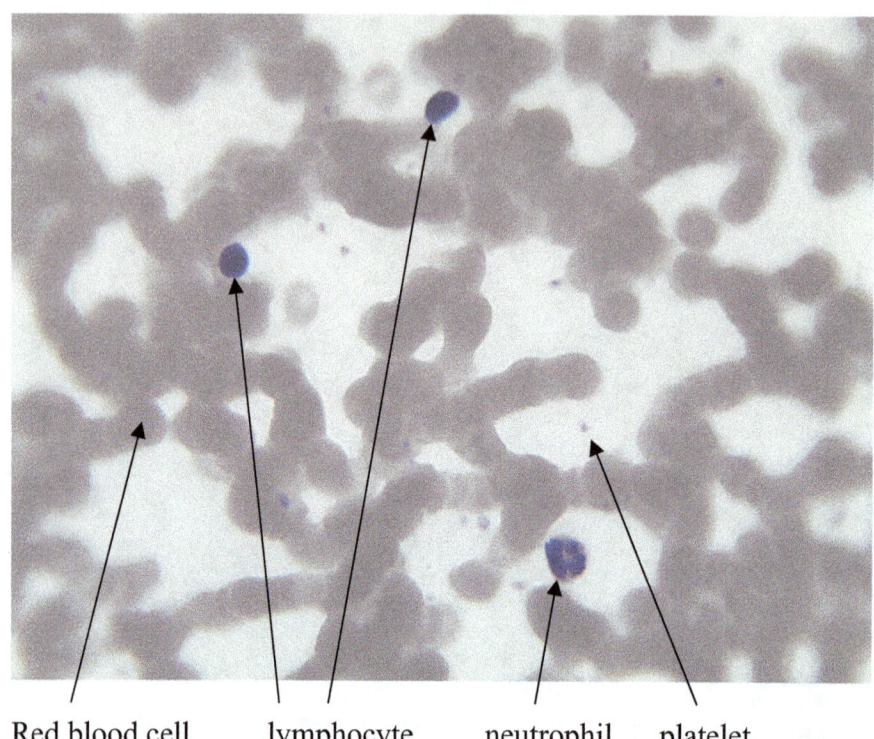

Red blood cell   lymphocyte   neutrophil   platelet

Blood at 1000X

Blood is a connective tissue and makes about 8% of our body weight.

Lymphocytes (WBC) are not much larger than a red blood cell and have a nucleus without lobes, which occupies most all of the cell.

Neutrophils are identified by the 3-5 lobes in the nucleus.

Platelets are just tiny fragments of cells and involved with clotting.

White blood cells come in 5 major groups: neutrophils, eosinophils, basophils, lymphocytes, monocytes.

BLOOD

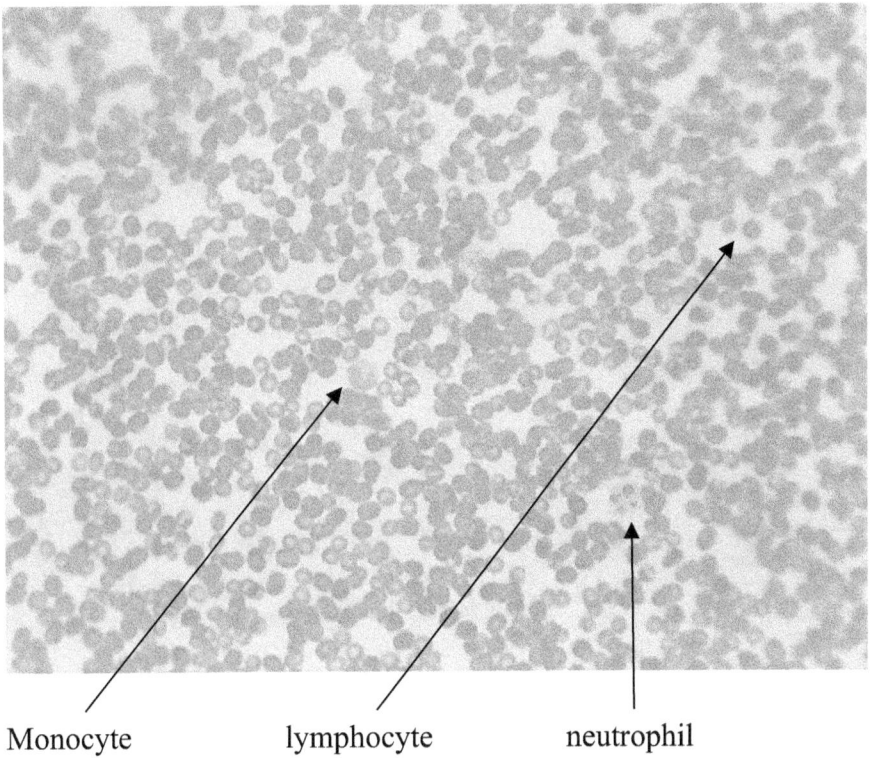

Monocyte   lymphocyte   neutrophil

Blood at 400X. Blood is a connective tissue.

The red blood cells are very numerous and easy to find and identify. White blood cells are scattered and fewer in number. The white blood cells are easy to find, due to the presence of the nucleus in each. Red blood cells don't have a nucleus in the mature form.

Monocytes are large white blood cells and often have a horseshoe shaped nucleus or a large round nucleus.

BLOOD (LEUKEMIA)

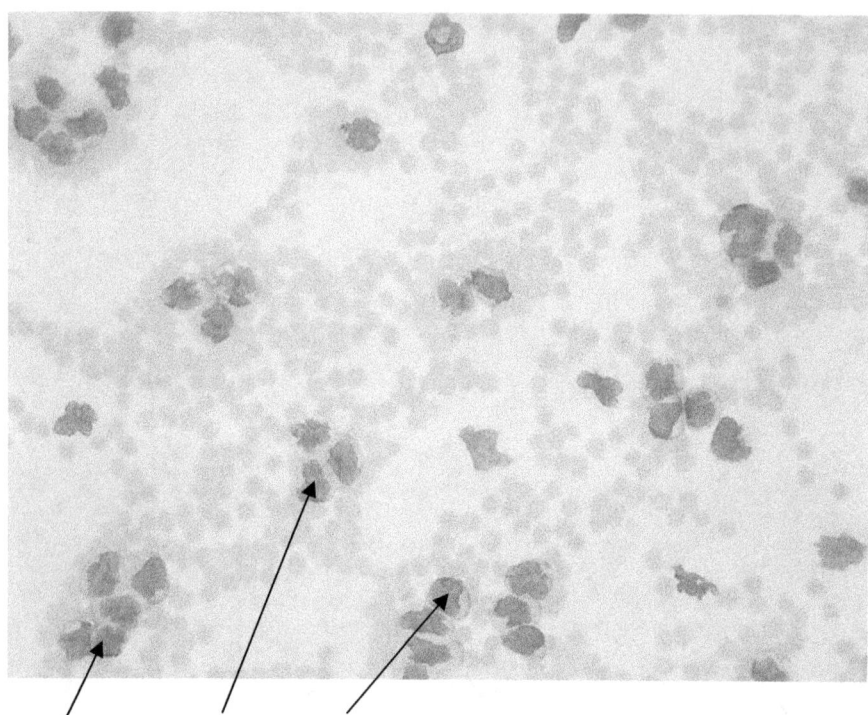

Abnormal white blood cells

Blood at 400X. Blood is a connective tissue.

Leukemia is a cancer of the blood and bone marrow.

Leukemia is characterized by a large number of abnormal white blood cells. These large, abnormal numbers will displace other healthy cells and result in problems such as anemia.

BLOOD (SICKLE CELL)

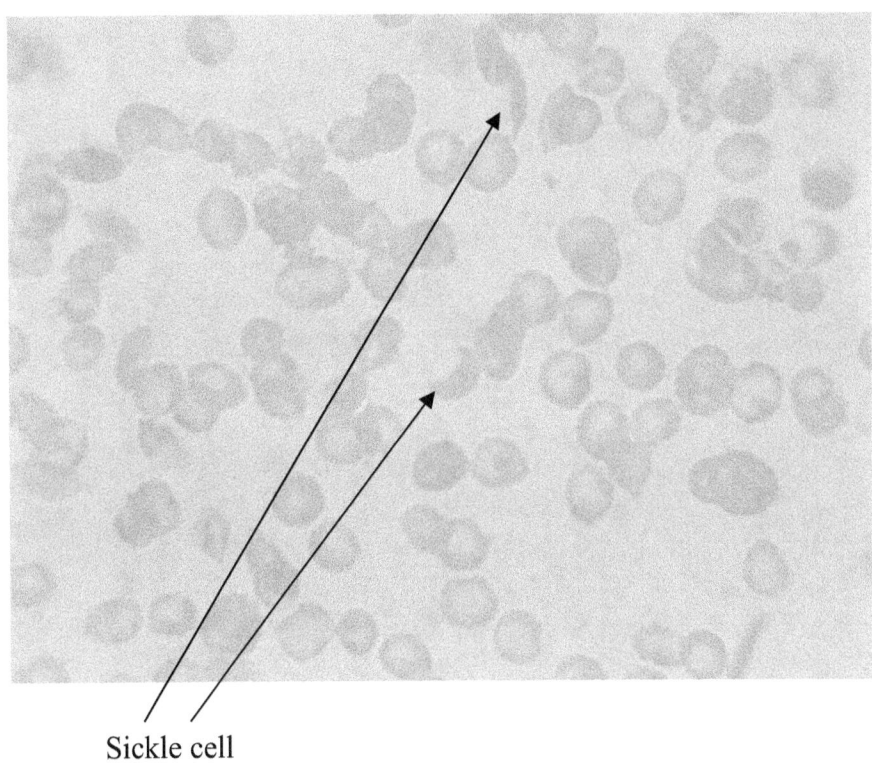

Sickle cell

Blood (sickle cell) at 1000X

When red blood cells take on a sickle (crescent moon) shape, they no longer bend and flex properly. When these cells reach a capillary, they no longer flex and pass through. This will stop blood flow and the tissue dies. Individuals with sickle cell anemia may suffer from strokes, heart attacks and a lack of blood flow to many other organs.

BLOOD (SICKLE CELL)

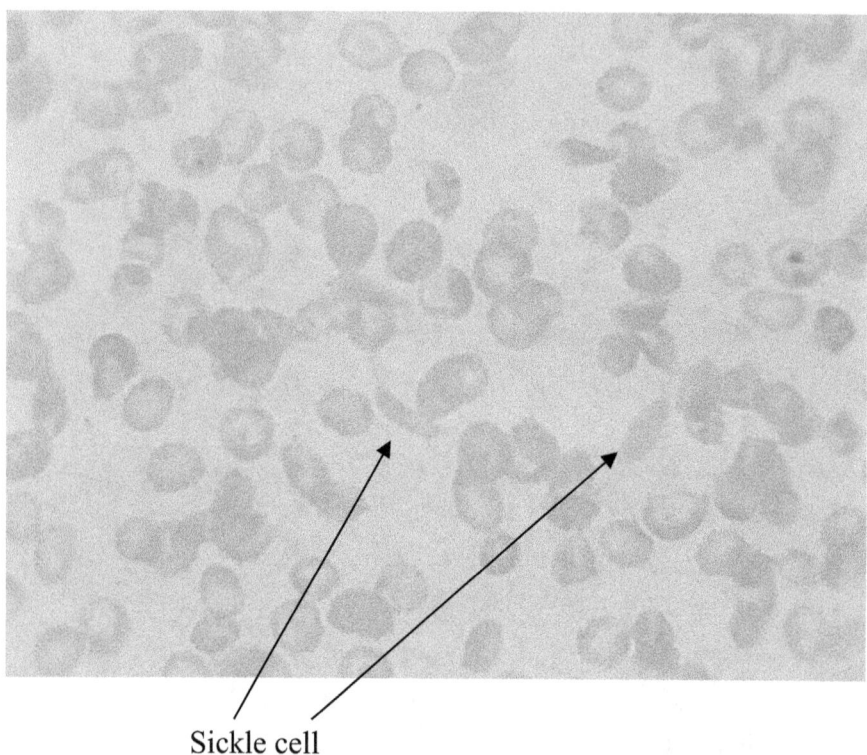

Sickle cell

Blood (sickle cell) at 1000X

Sickle cell anemia is an adaptation to individuals being exposed to malaria over many generations. The malaria parasite needs a normal round biconcave red blood cell to infect. A sickle shaped cell can't be infected, but it won't bend and flex properly.

BONE MARROW

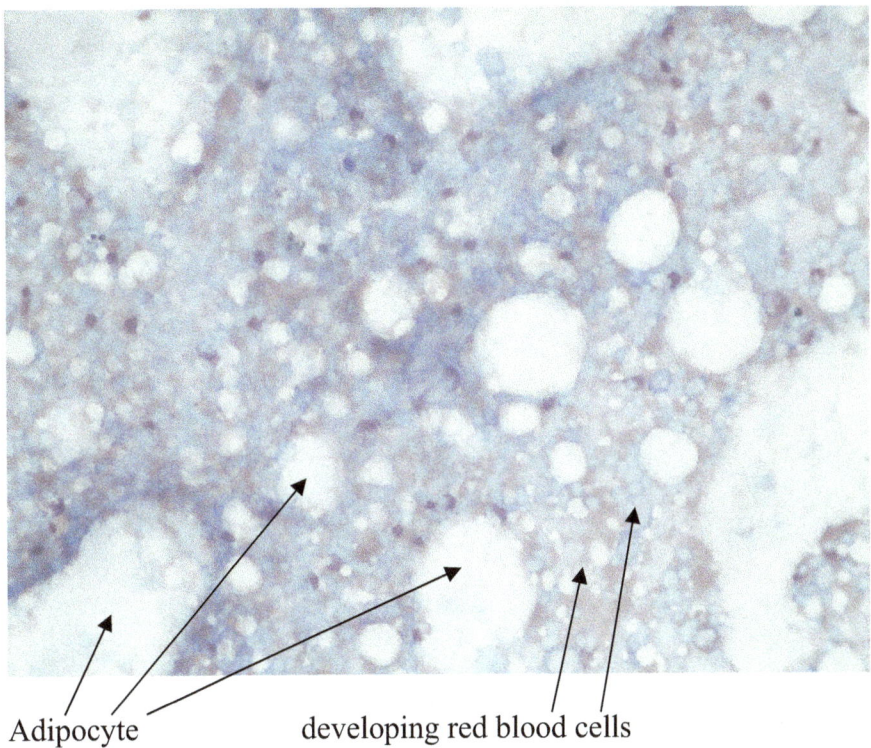

Adipocyte   developing red blood cells

Bone marrow at 40X. Bone marrow is a connective tissue.

The bone marrow is also called hemopoietic tissue. This is where the cells of the blood are developing.

The bone marrow is found within the large bones of our body.

The bone marrow is where all of the cells of the blood (formed elements) are produced.

Bone marrow comes in 2 forms, red and yellow. Red bone marrow is also called young bone marrow. Yellow bone marrow is also called adult bone marrow. The only big difference between the 2 is that we have more adipocytes in adult marrow. Yellow bone marrow is pictured above, notice all the fat cells.

BONE MARROW

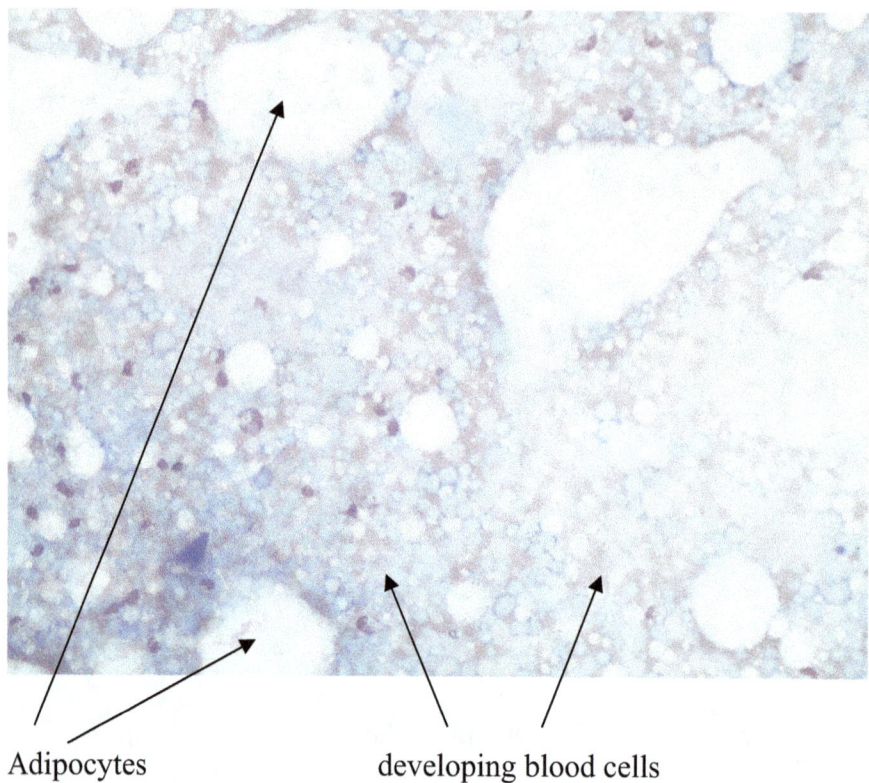

Adipocytes   developing blood cells

Bone marrow at 40X. Bone marrow is a connective tissue.

The bone marrow is where the cells of the blood are formed. Red blood cells, white blood cells and platelets are formed here.
There are two types of bone marrow, red and yellow. When we are young our marrow is of the red type and has a small amount of fat cells (adipocytes) in it. As we get older, we don't have such a demand for red blood cell production and adipose tissue replaces some of the stem cells producing the cells of the blood.
Hemopoietic tissue is another name for the tissue producing the cells of the blood.

CANCELLOUS BONE

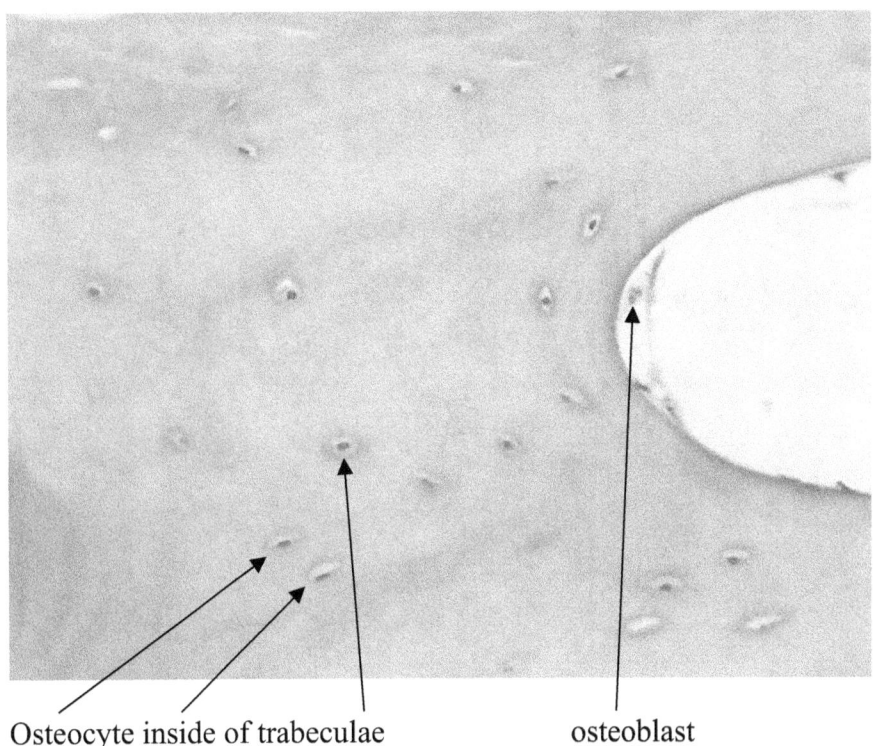

Osteocyte inside of trabeculae   osteoblast

Cancellous bone at 400X. Bone is a connective tissue.

Cancellous bone is also called spongy bone. This bone is not soft like a sponge, but it has interconnecting pieces called trabeculae that make this type of bone look like a sponge.

Osteocytes are cells that maintain the bone, osteoblasts are cells which build bone and osteoclasts break down bone.

CARDIAC MUSCLE

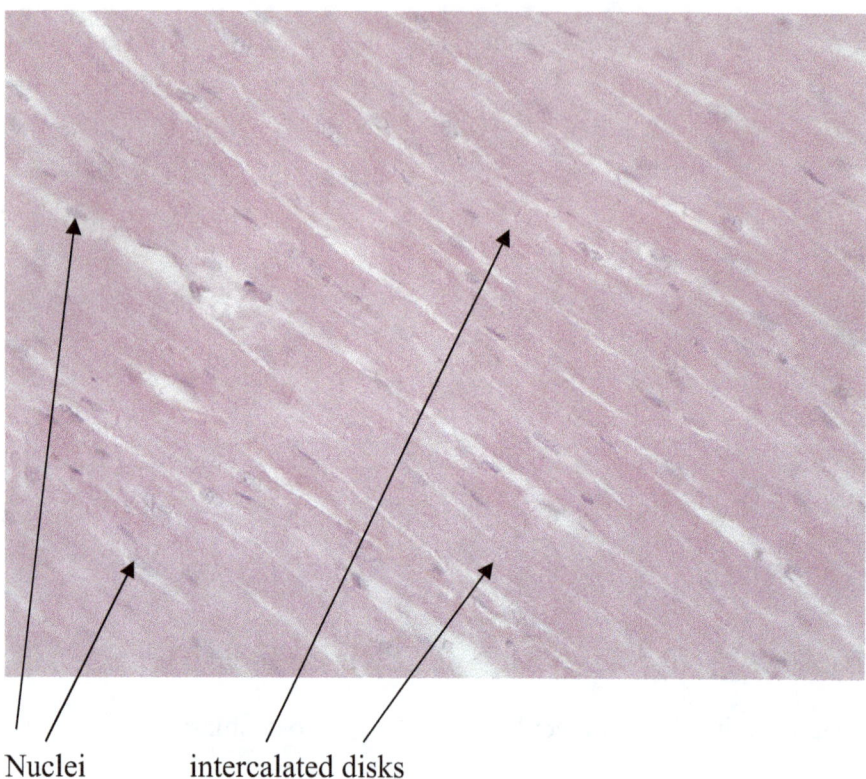

Nuclei   intercalated disks

Cardiac muscle at 400X

Cardiac muscle is only found in the heart.

Cardiac muscle has a cylinder shape with connections between the cells. The cells are striated but the striations (stripes) are often difficult to see. Intercalated disks are junctions seen between cells and only seen in this muscle type. Cardiac muscle is involuntary and usually has one centrally located nucleus.

CARDIAC MUSCLE

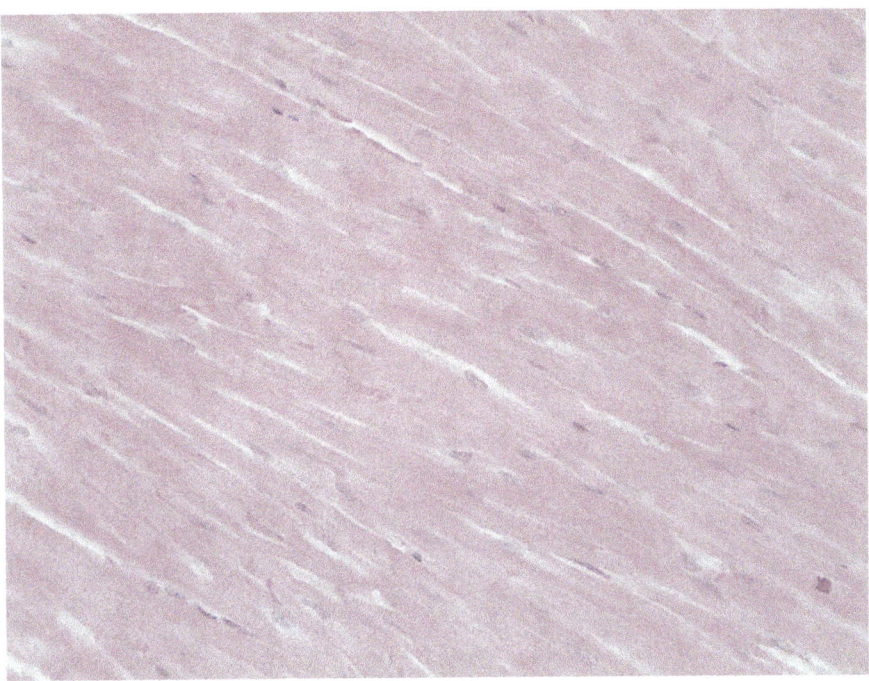

Cardiac muscle at 400X

Cardiac muscle comprises most all of the heart and is the main force responsible for generating the pressure which moves our blood.

The cardiac muscle receives oxygen rich blood through several large arteries. The coronary, marginal and interventricular are just a few of these arteries. If the cardiac muscle becomes oxygen deprived for more than 20 minutes the cells will die. This is what we call a myocardial infarction, meaning an area of cell death among the myocardium or heart attack. Muscle cells are made during embryonic development, so once they are lost, they can't be replaced.

CARDIAC MUSCLE

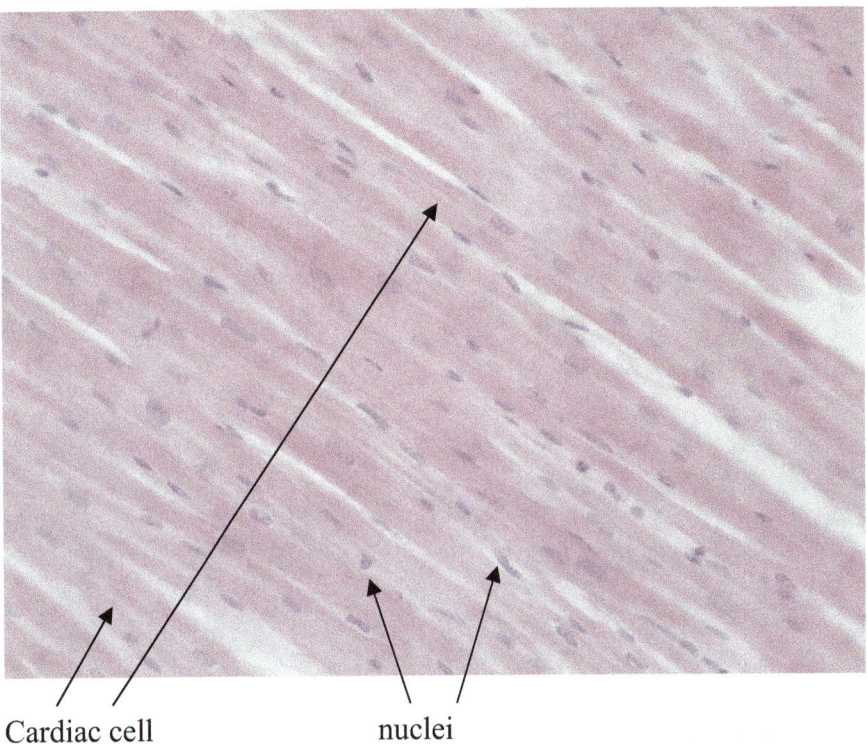

Cardiac cell   nuclei

Cardiac muscle at 400X

Action potentials (electric signals) travel through cardiac muscle slower than they do in skeletal muscle. The action potentials travel slower because of the smaller diameter of cardiac muscle cells and through the use of more calcium channels. We want cardiac muscle to contact slower, because a slow forceful contraction will push more blood than a rapid contraction.

CARDIAC MUSCLE

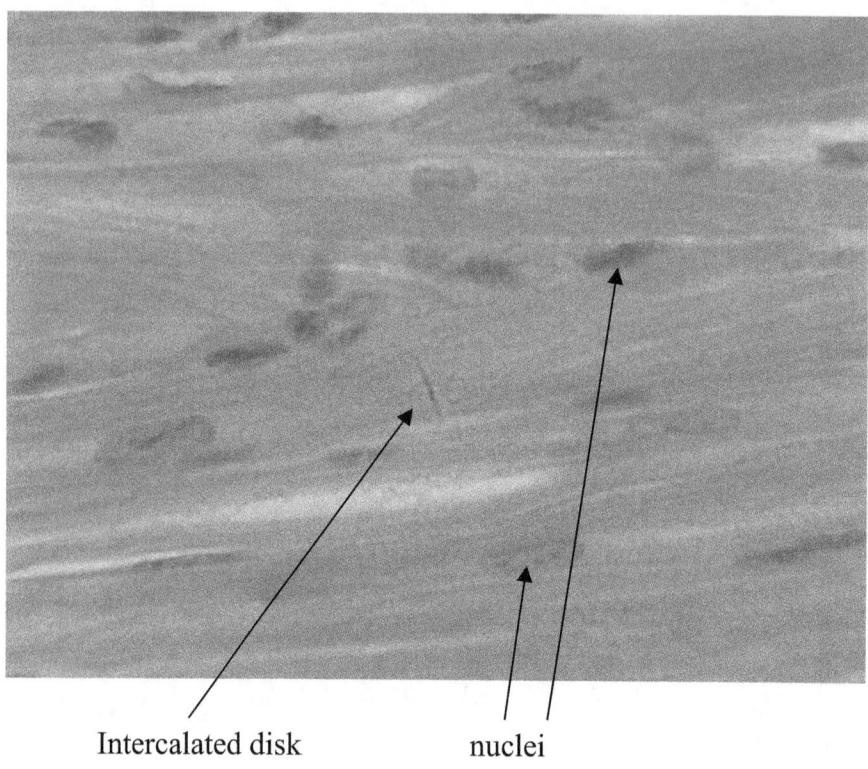

Intercalated disk   nuclei

Cardiac muscle at 1000X

CEREBELLUM

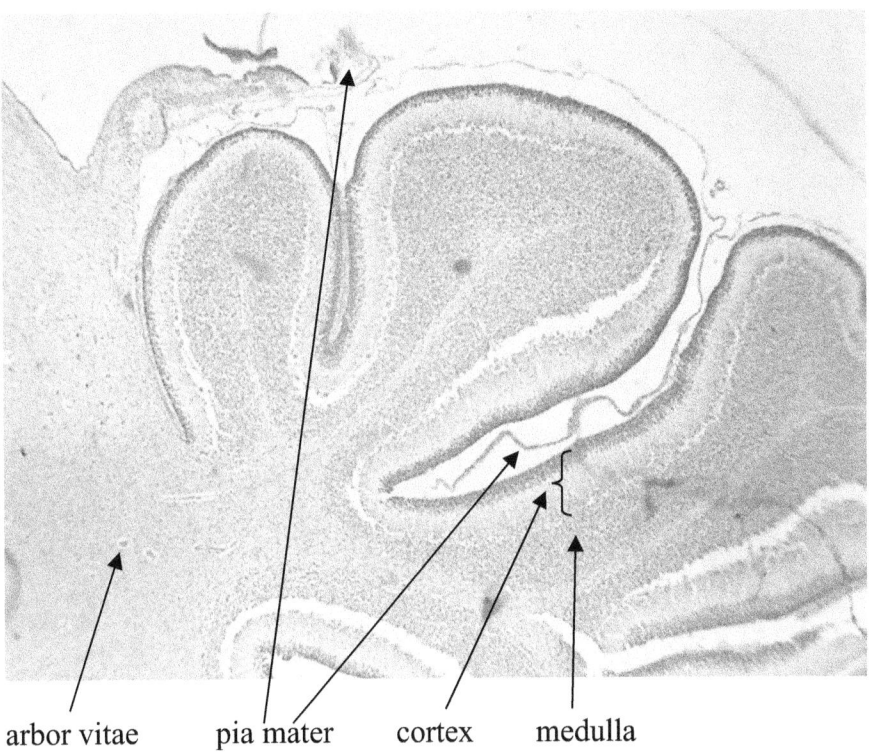

arbor vitae   pia mater   cortex   medulla

Cerebellum at 40X. The cerebellum is nervous tissue.

Folia – the ridges seen on the cerebellum.

The arbor vitae is the mylineated (white matter) area where axons are found.

The pia mater is the deepest of the meninges and is found attached to the surface of the brain.

Cortex is always an outer region and medulla is always an inner region.

CEREBELLUM

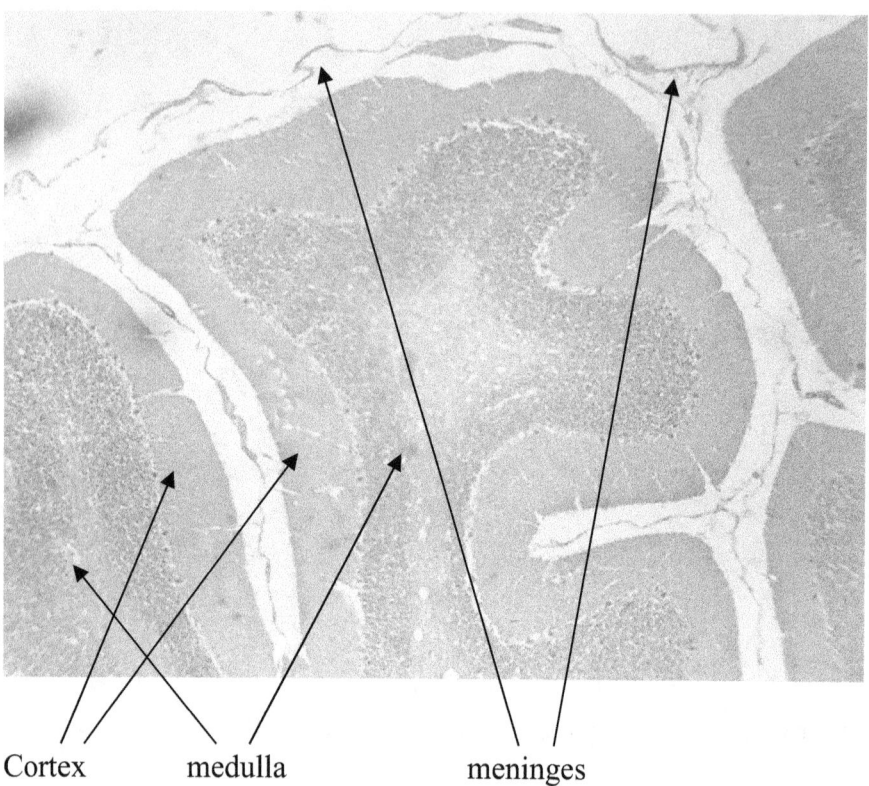

Cortex   medulla   meninges

Cerebellum at 40X

The outer cortex is composed of grey matter, consisting of neuron cell bodies and dendrites.

The deeper inner medulla is composed of mylineated axons.

The cerebellum is the small part of the brain to the rear of the skull behind the occipital bone.

This part of the brain is responsible for muscle movement, muscle coordination and balance.

CEREBELLUM

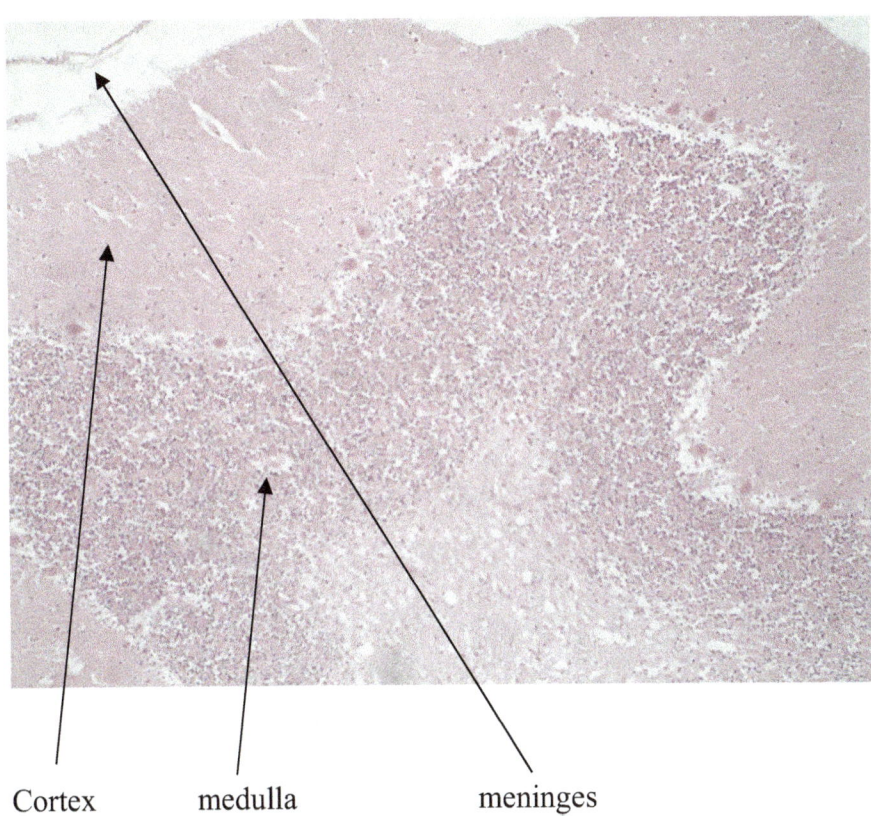

Cortex   medulla   meninges

Cerebellum at 100X

The cerebellum is an incredibly complex part of the brain, and many functions are found here. One function is the learning of complex movements. We can move our body is smooth fluid movements because of this part of the brain.

The cerebellum has three major regions to it: the lateral hemispheres, the vermis and the flocculonodular lobes.

CEREBELLUM

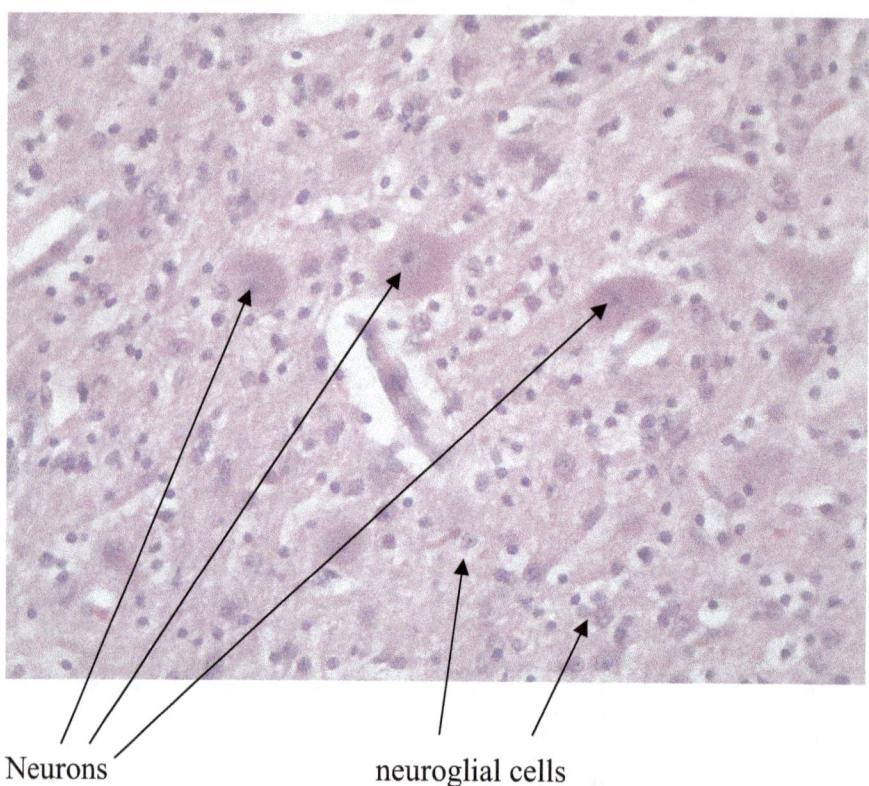

Neurons   neuroglial cells

Cerebellum at 400X

Neurons and many neuroglial cells can be seen at 400X. Neuroglial cells are supporting cells of the nervous system. These cells are much more numerous than neurons but are much smaller.

CEREBRUM

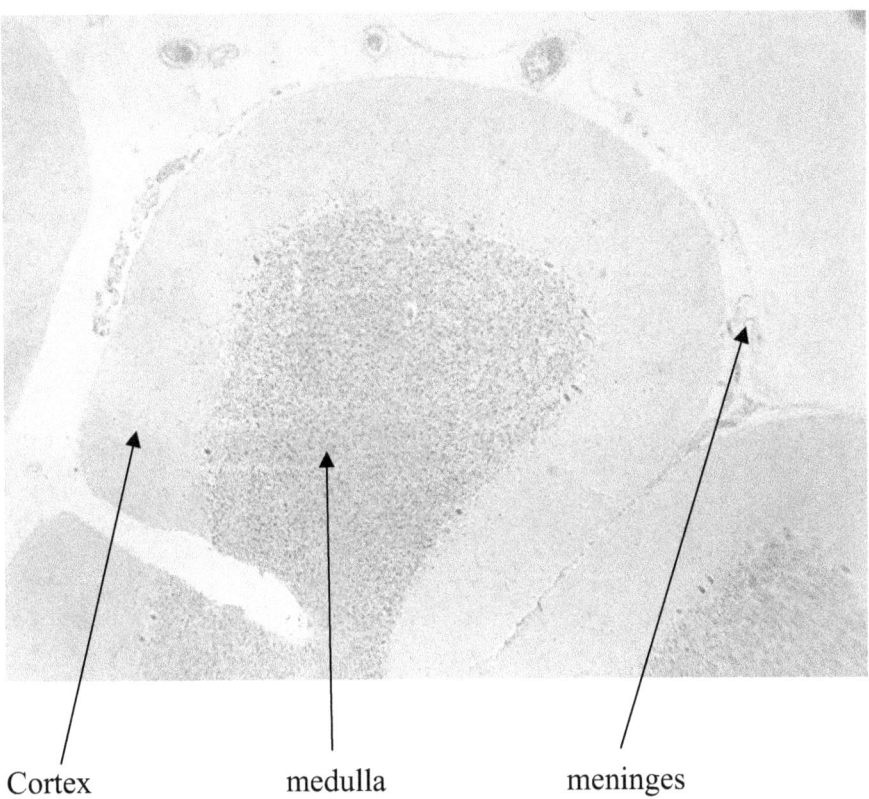

Cortex   medulla   meninges

Cerebrum at 40X

The outer cortex is composed of grey matter, consisting of neuron cell bodies and dendrites.

The deeper inner medulla is composed of mylineated axons.

The cerebrum is the largest part of the brain, consisting of 2 hemispheres and 4 lobes.

The cerebrum has many functions. Some of these functions include voluntary movement, emotions, mood, memory, smell, hearing and vision.

CEREBRUM

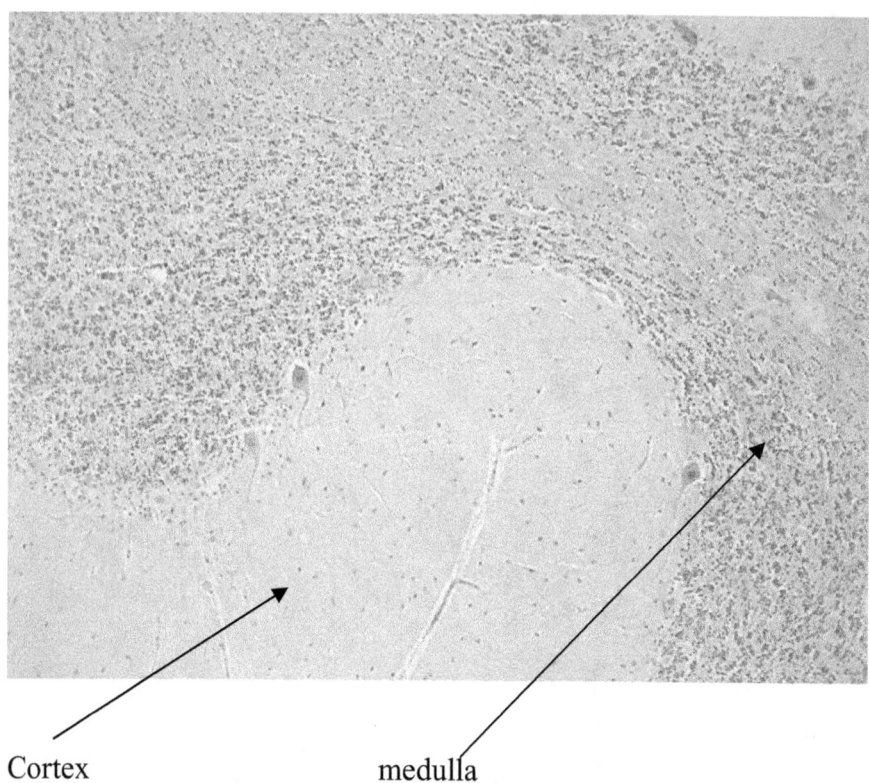

Cortex   medulla

Cerebrum at 100X

The cerebrum forms the bulk of the brain and is divided into two large hemispheres. Each hemisphere of the cerebrum is divided out into lobes.

The cerebrum has many functions. Some of these functions includes conscious perception, voluntary motor function, memory and thoughts.

CEREBRUM

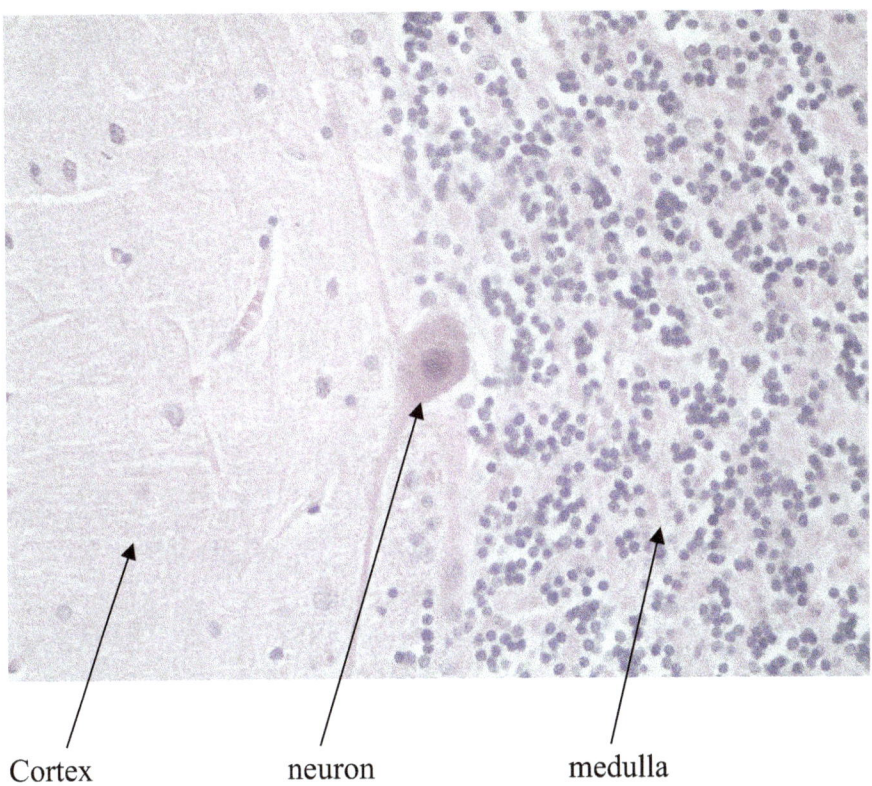

Cortex   neuron   medulla

Cerebrum at 400X

Notice how large the neurons are in comparison to the neuroglial cells. The neuroglial cells are smaller, but they are much more numerous than neurons.

CERVIX

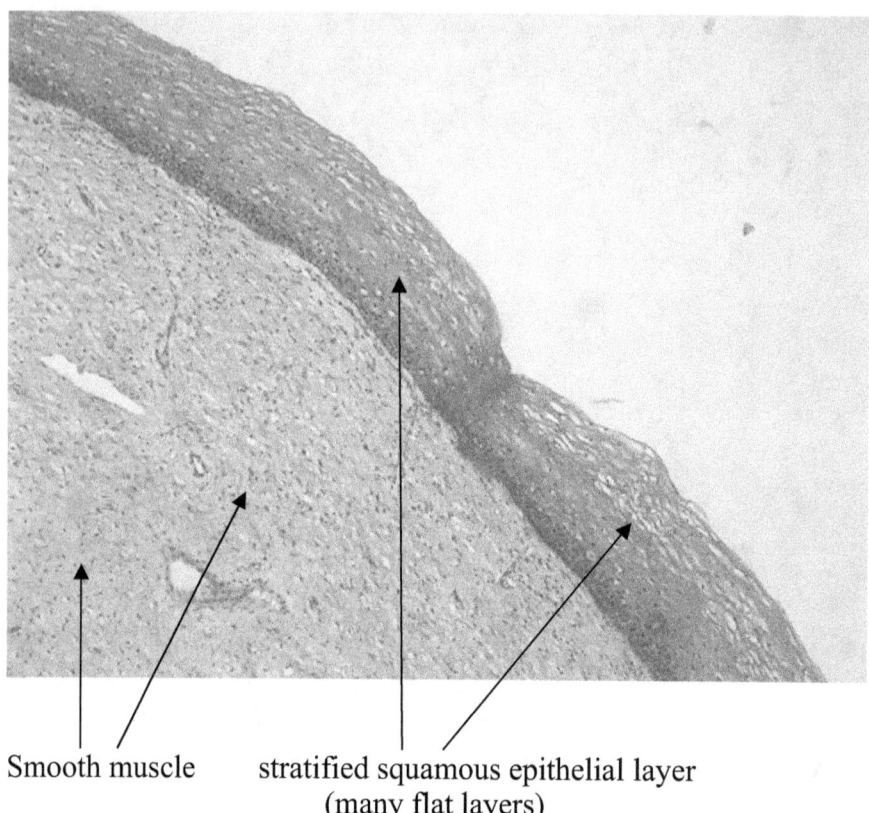

Smooth muscle   stratified squamous epithelial layer
(many flat layers)

Cervix at 100X

The cervix is the inferior, narrowed part of the uterus. The cervix is one part of the uterus. The uterus is a hollow, muscular organ in which the baby grows and develops.

The endometrium is the inner layer of the uterus that builds up every month for the preparation of implantation. If a pregnancy doesn't occur this inner layer is removed and rebuilds.

The smooth muscle of the uterus will contract in response to the hormone oxytocin. This hormone will cause the labor contractions, responsible for the expelling of the baby.

CERVIX

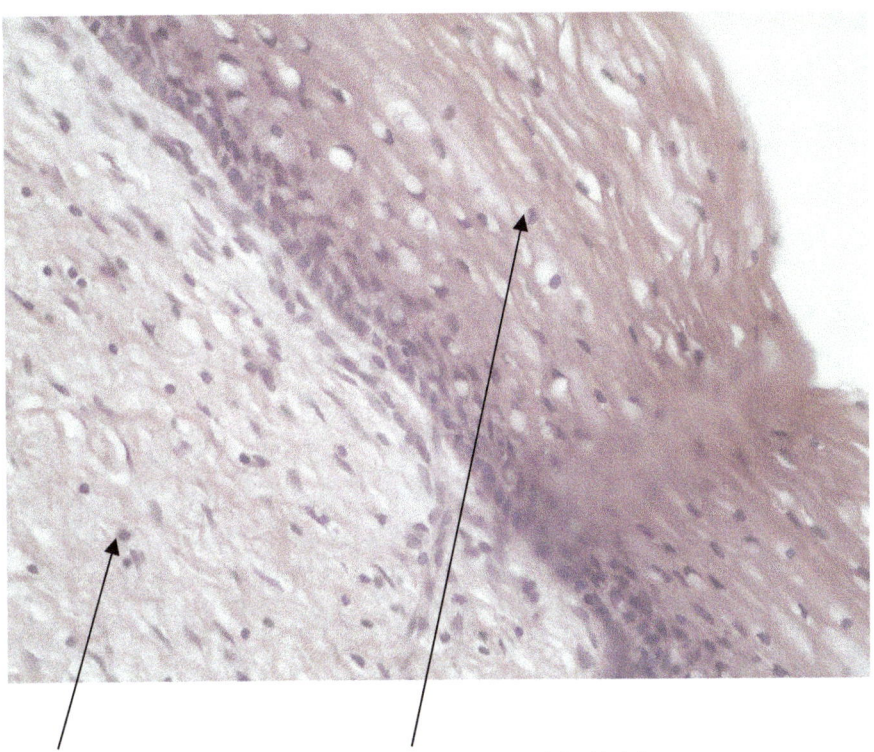

Smooth muscle   stratified squamous epithelial layer
                 (many flat layers)

Cervix at 400X

The endometrium is the inner layer of the uterus that builds up every month for the preparation of implantation. If a pregnancy doesn't occur this inner layer is removed and rebuilds.

The smooth muscle of the uterus will contract in response to the hormone oxytocin. This hormone will cause the labor contractions, responsible for the expelling of the baby.

CHROMOSOMES

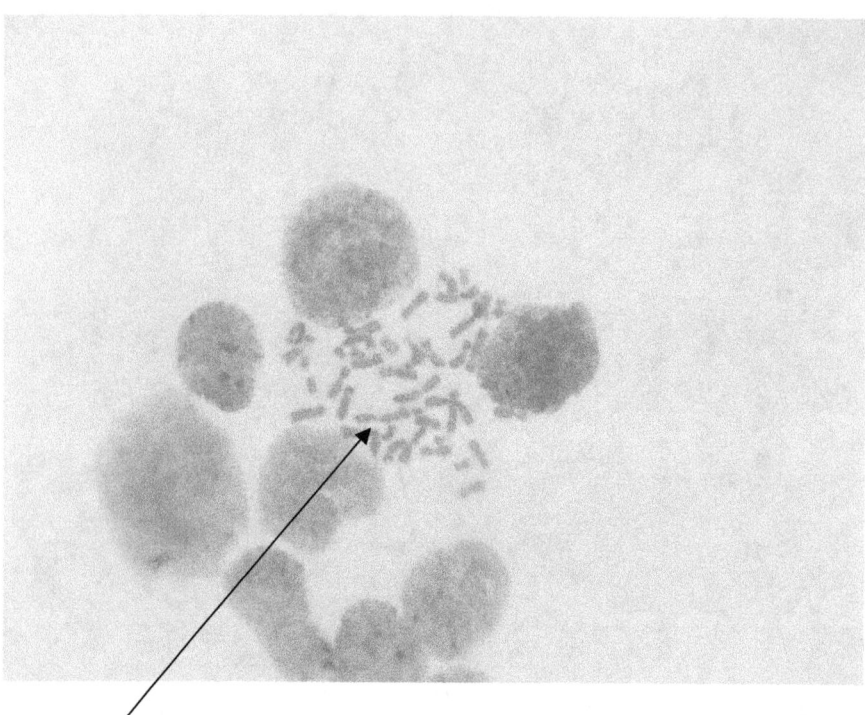

Chromosomes at 1000X

Humans have 23 pairs of chromosomes.

Each chromosome is made up of two pairs of chromatids, connected together by a centromere. Chromosomes are the organized material we call DNA. DNA is usually found in the form of chromatin. When a cell leaves interphase and enters prophase, the chromatin will condense into the compact chromosome form.

CHROMOSOMES

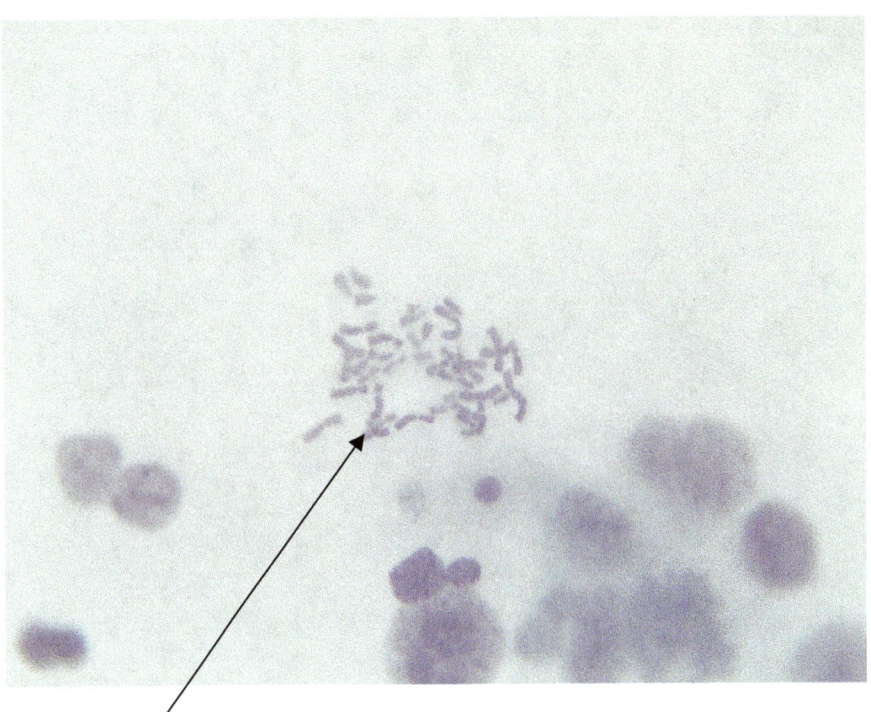

Chromosomes at 1000X

Humans have 23 pairs of chromosomes in all cells except the reproductive cells (haploid cells).

CILIATED PSEUDOSTRATIFIED

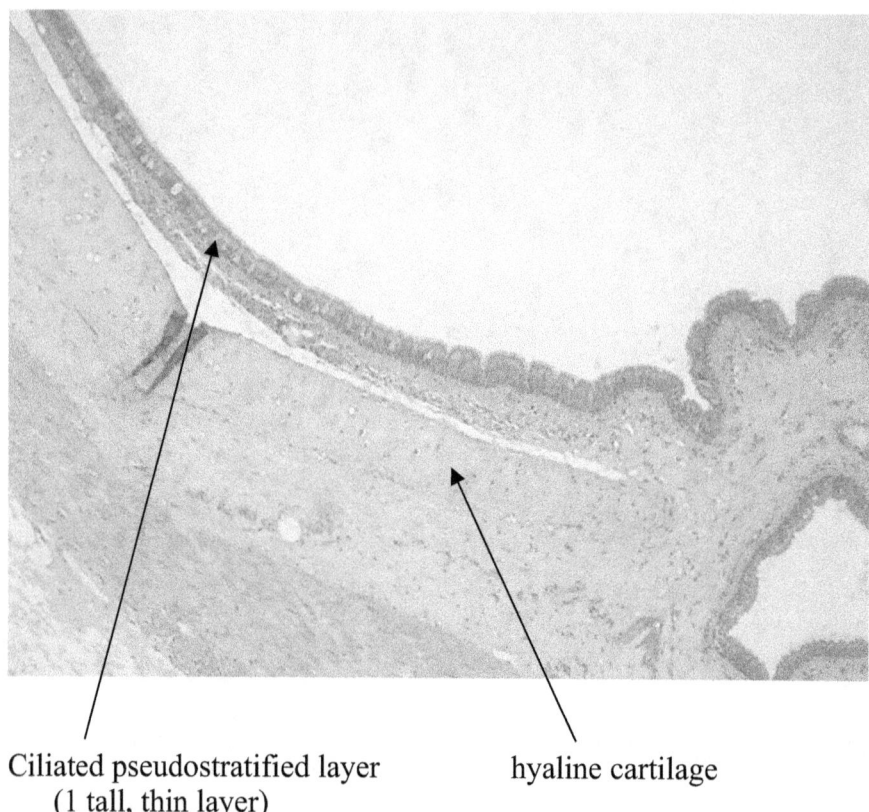

Ciliated pseudostratified layer　　　hyaline cartilage
 (1 tall, thin layer)

Ciliated Pseudostratified at 100X

Ciliated pseudostratified is an epithelial tissue.

Cilia are used by cells to move materials over their surface. Cilia are often found moving mucous, but other materials like oocytes may be moved also.

CILIATED PSEUDOSTRATIFIED

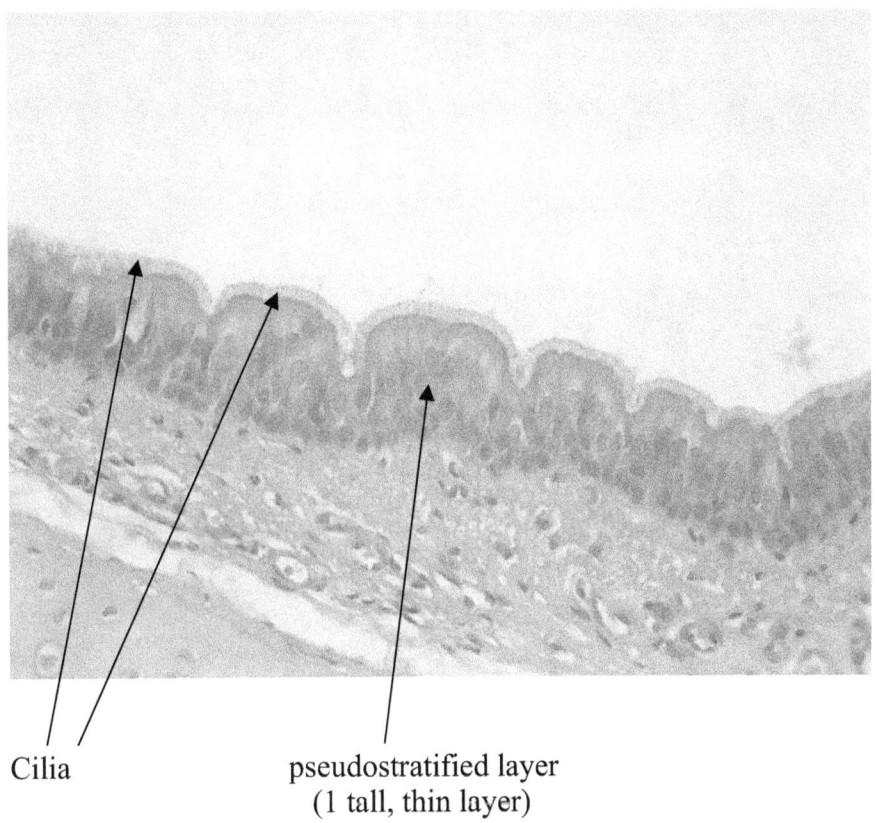

Cilia

pseudostratified layer
(1 tall, thin layer)

Ciliated Pseudostratified at 400X

Notice how the cilia always look like a fuzzy border.

This ciliated pseudostratified layer was taken from the trachea.

CILIATED PSEUDOSTRATIFIED

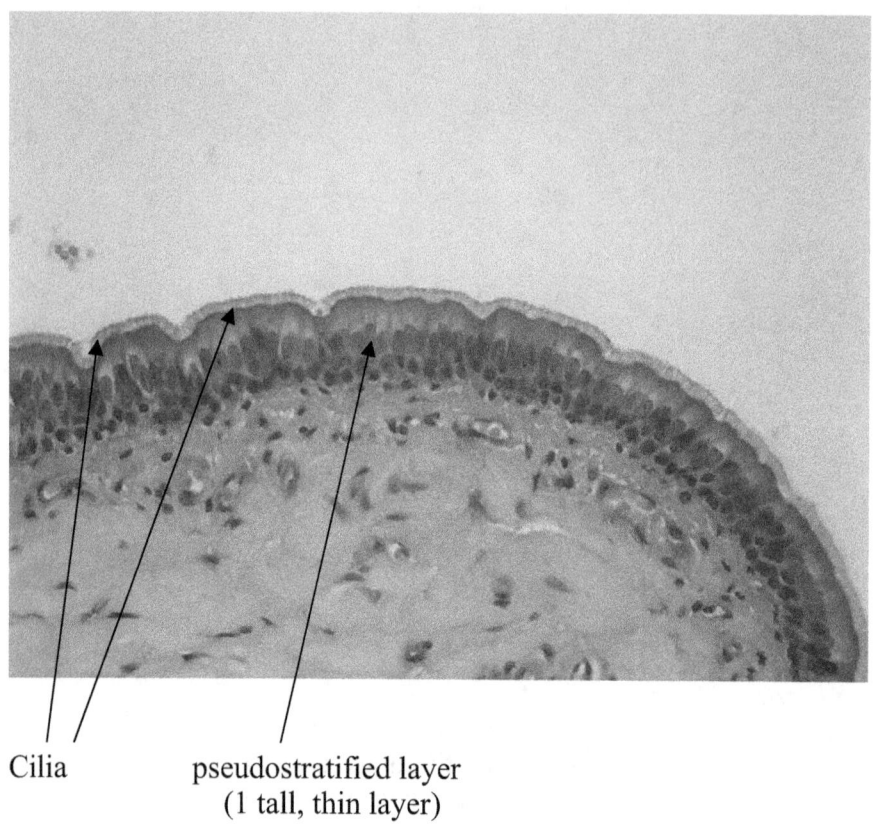

Cilia   pseudostratified layer
        (1 tall, thin layer)

Ciliated Pseudostratified at 400X

The nuclei of the pseudostratified layer are easily seen. These nuclei often look elongated and that is what makes a pseudostratified layer easily identifiable.

COCHLEA

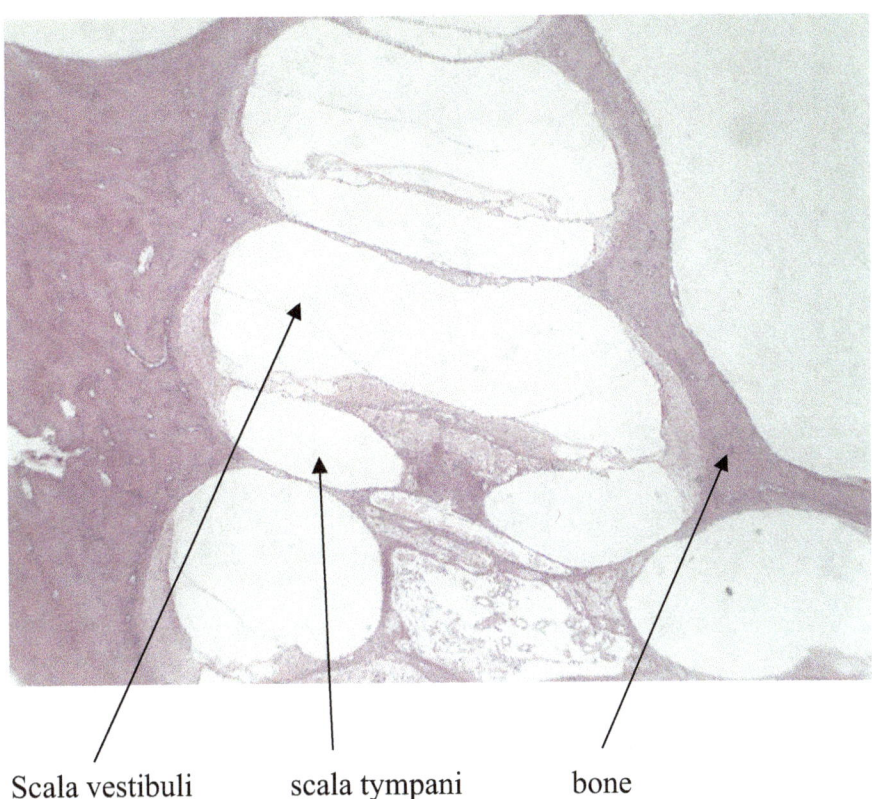

Scala vestibuli   scala tympani   bone

Cochlea at 40X

The cochlea is a spiral organ deep inside the inner ear and responsible for hearing. The cochlea is surrounded by bone and the inner chambers are filled with lymphs (fluids) and sensory structures.

COLON

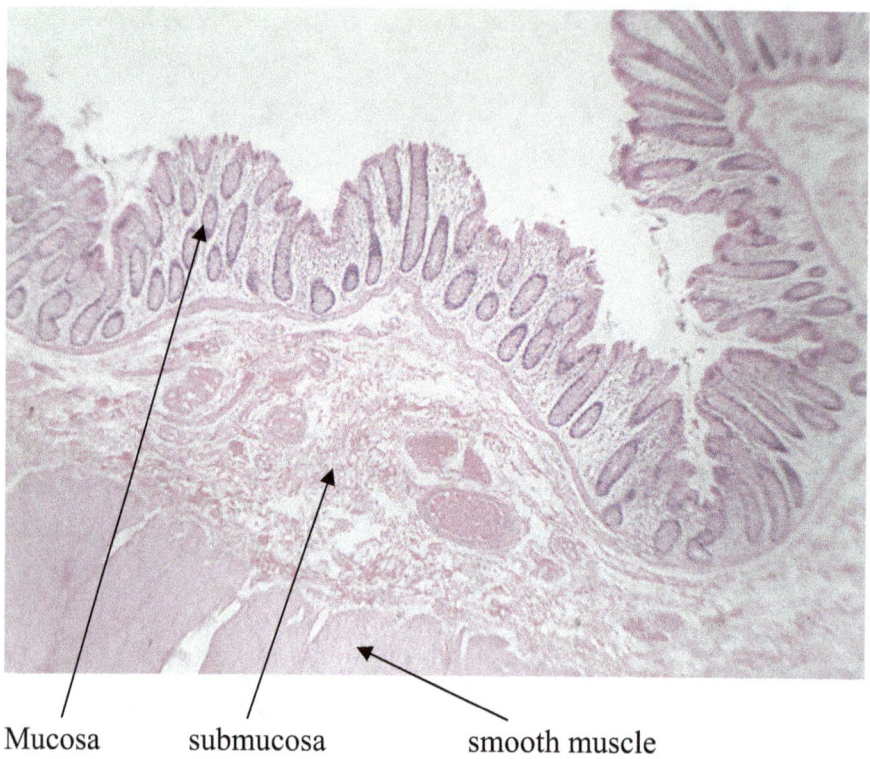

Mucosa   submucosa   smooth muscle

Colon at 40X

The colon is the largest part of the large intestine. In the large intestine most of the remaining water is reabsorbed back into the body. The contractions of the smooth muscle in this area is referred to as mass movements.

The large intestine contains many helpful microorganisms, and we enjoy a nice symbiotic relationship with them. One of the helpful materials bacteria in the large intestine make for us is vitamin K. The action of bacteria in the large intestine produces a gas we call flatus.

COLON

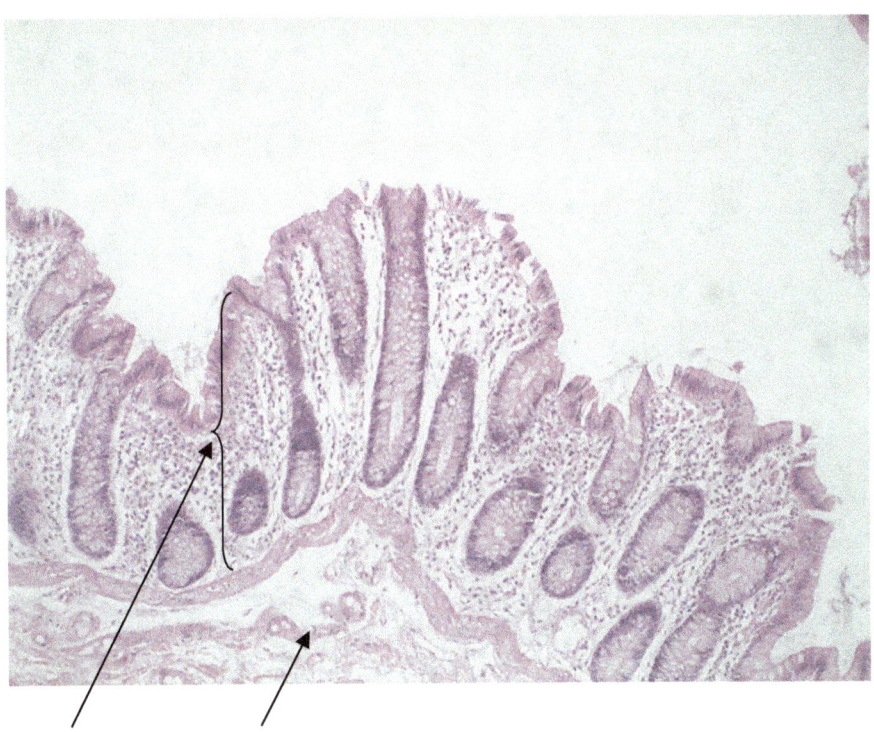

Mucosa   submucosa

Colon at 100X

The glands and the goblet cells of the colon start to appear as we magnify up to 100X.

Along the large intestine are many small segments which look like pouches. These pouches are called haustra. Haustra can't be seen in a slide, they are much too large.

COLON

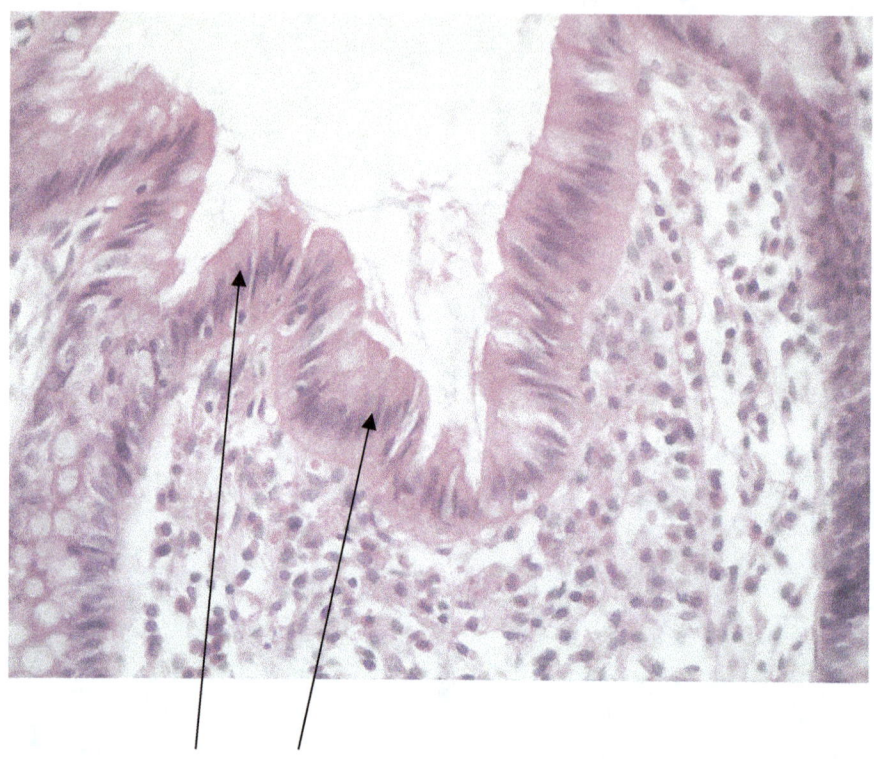

Simple columnar cell layer (epithelial tissue)
(1 tall, thin layer)

Colon at 400X

The tall thin layer of epithelial tissue comes into focus at 400X.

The large intestine has many fatty deposits on its superficial surface. These deposits are called epiploic appendages.

As the cells of the large intestine reabsorb most of the remaining water, the remaining material will leave the body as what we call feces.

COMPACT BONE

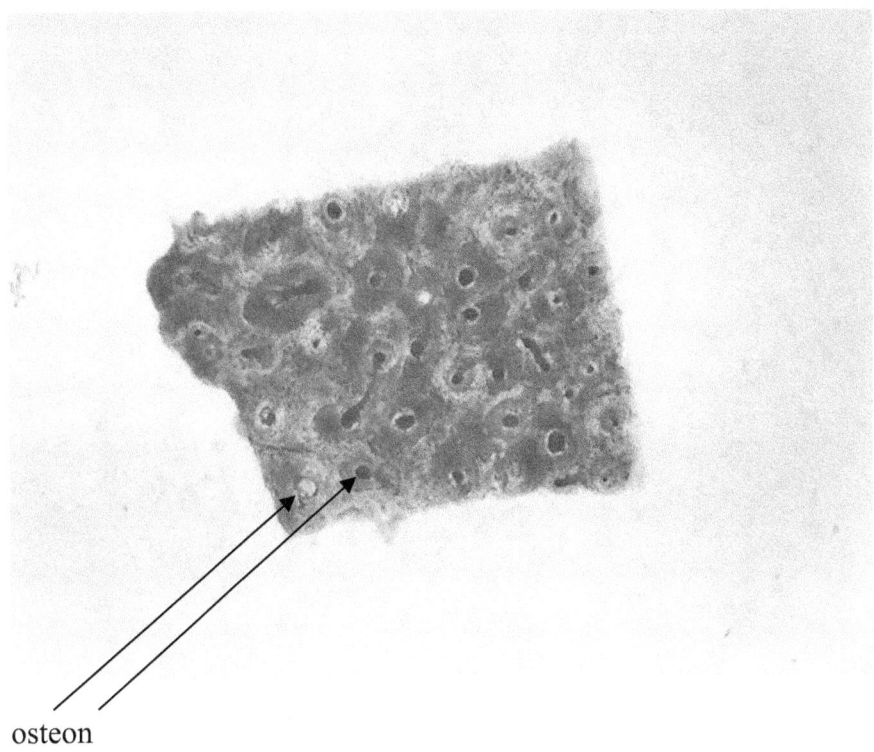

osteon

Bone at 40X. Compact bone is a connective tissue.

Notice all of the osteons seen in bone. Osteons are also called Haversian systems and they are the functional units of bone.

No other tissue in the human body has an appearance like hard, compact bone. Compact bone is used for support and protection. Our bones support the other tissues and make the general shape of our body. Compact bone protects deeper softer structures in the body. Our skull protects our brain, and the sternum and ribs protect the heart and lungs.

COMPACT BONE

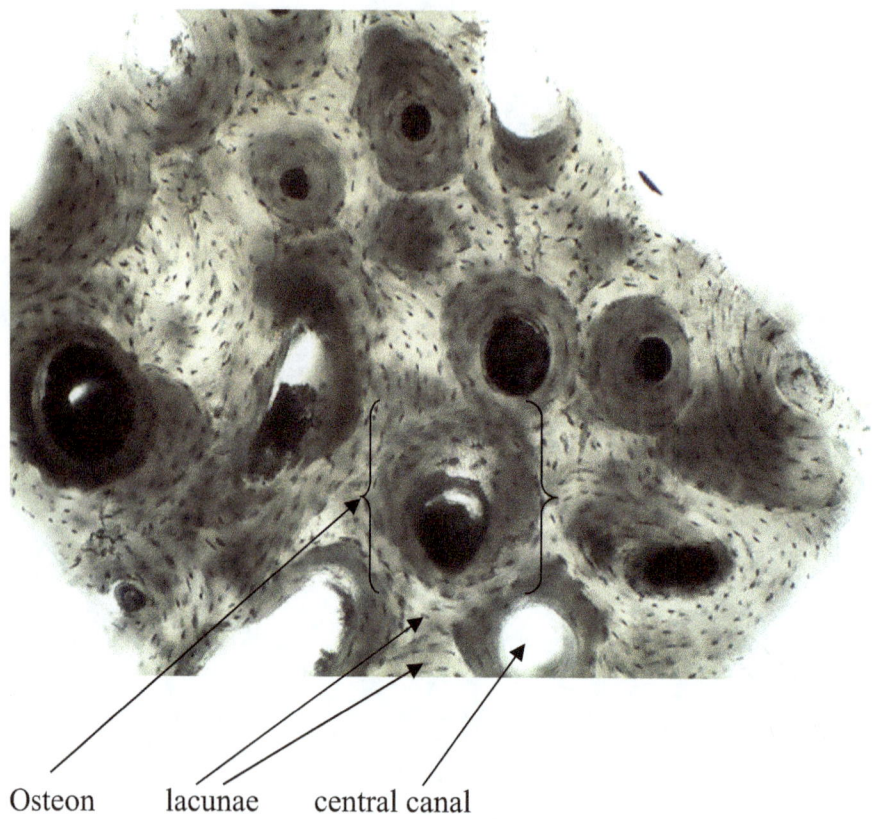

Osteon   lacunae   central canal

Bone at 100X. Compact bone is a connective tissue.

Each osteon looks like a tree stump. Nothing else looks like compact bone.

All of the tiny dark dots you see are lacunae. The lacunae are hollow spaces within the bone matrix, where osteocytes live.

The central canal is where a tiny artery and vein would be found.

COMPACT BONE

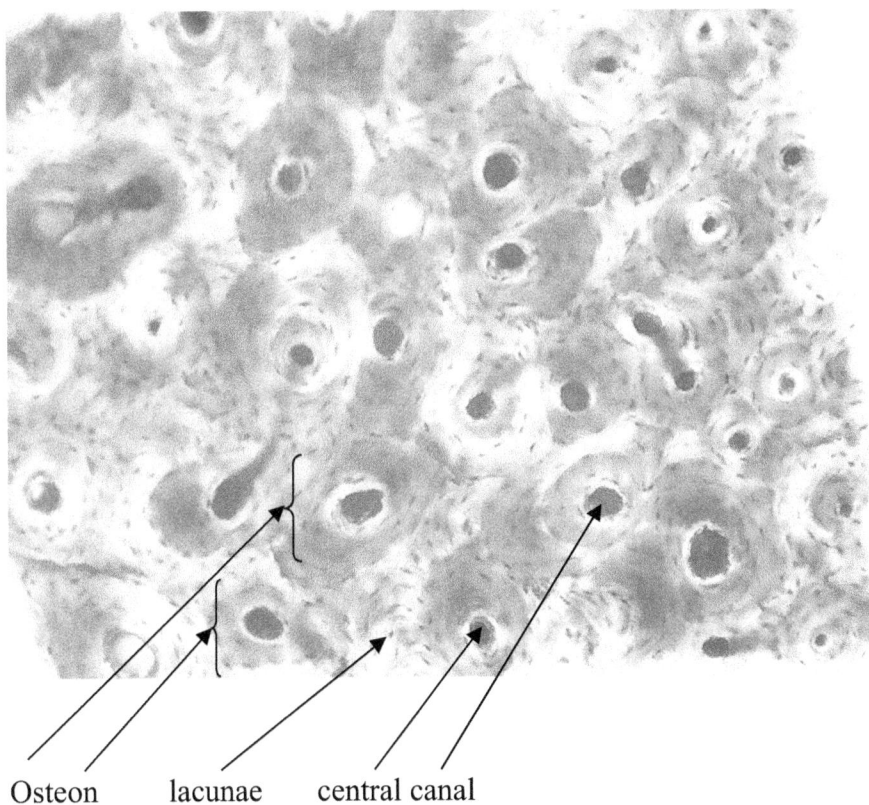

Osteon   lacunae   central canal

Bone at 100X. Compact bone is a connective tissue.

Bone contains three main cell types: osteoblasts (build bone), osteoclasts (break down bone) and osteocytes (maintain bone).

Bone matrix is largely made of two materials collagen and hydroxyapatite. Collagen gives bone flexibility and hydroxyapatite gives bone its hard, weight bearing strength.

Inside each osteon is a set of rings, one inside of another. Each one of these rings is called a concentric lamellae.

DIAPHRAGM MUSCLE

Diaphragm muscle at 400X

The diaphragm is a thin layer of skeletal muscle which separates the thoracic and abdominal cavities.

This muscle is used in the process of ventilation, which is the movement of air in and out of the lungs.

When relaxed this muscle is in a superior position and dome shaped. When the muscle contracts it moves in an inferior direction. As the diaphragm contracts, it increases the volume of the thoracic cavity. As the volume of the thoracic cavity increases the pressure inside decreases. This will move air into the lungs. This change in volume and pressure is called Boyle's Law.

ELASTIC TISSUE

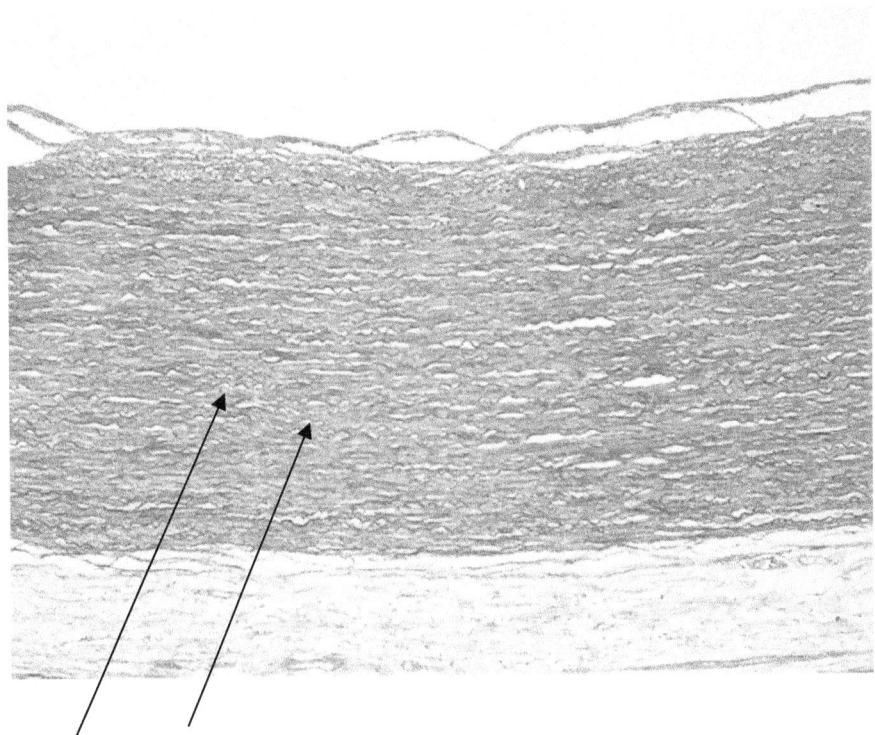

Elastic tissue filled with elastic fibers.

Elastic tissue at 100X

Elastic fibers stain dark on a histology slide. If you see a dark stain like this one and can see the lines of dark fibers, then elastic fibers are probably present.

Elastic tissue is found where we need tissues to stretch. These fibers are like rubber bands.

This slide is from an artery. Arteries contain large amounts of elastic tissue, so they will stretch. This stretching helps to stabilize our blood pressure. As we get older, we lose these elastic fibers and our arteries harden.

ELASTIC TISSUE

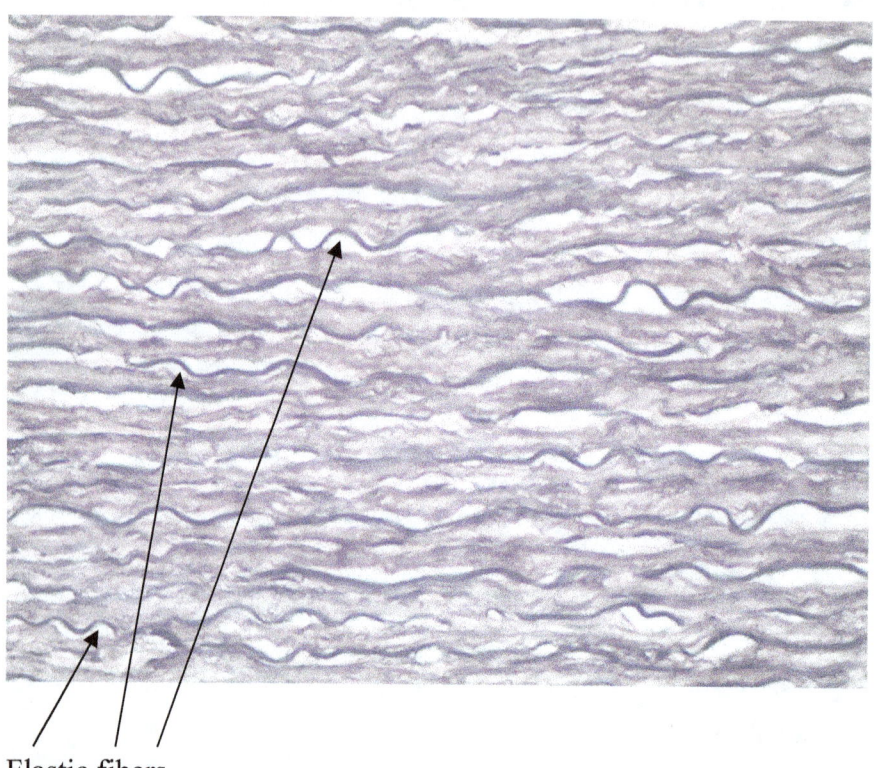

Elastic fibers

Elastic tissue at 400X

Elastic tissue stretches easily and is found in great abundance in arteries. As we age, we lose the elastic fibers and arteries will harden.

Elastic fibers stain dark on a histology slide. If you see a dark stain like this one and can see the lines of dark fibers, then elastic fibers are probably present.

Elastic tissue is found where we need tissues to stretch. These fibers are like rubber bands.

ELASTIC CARTILAGE

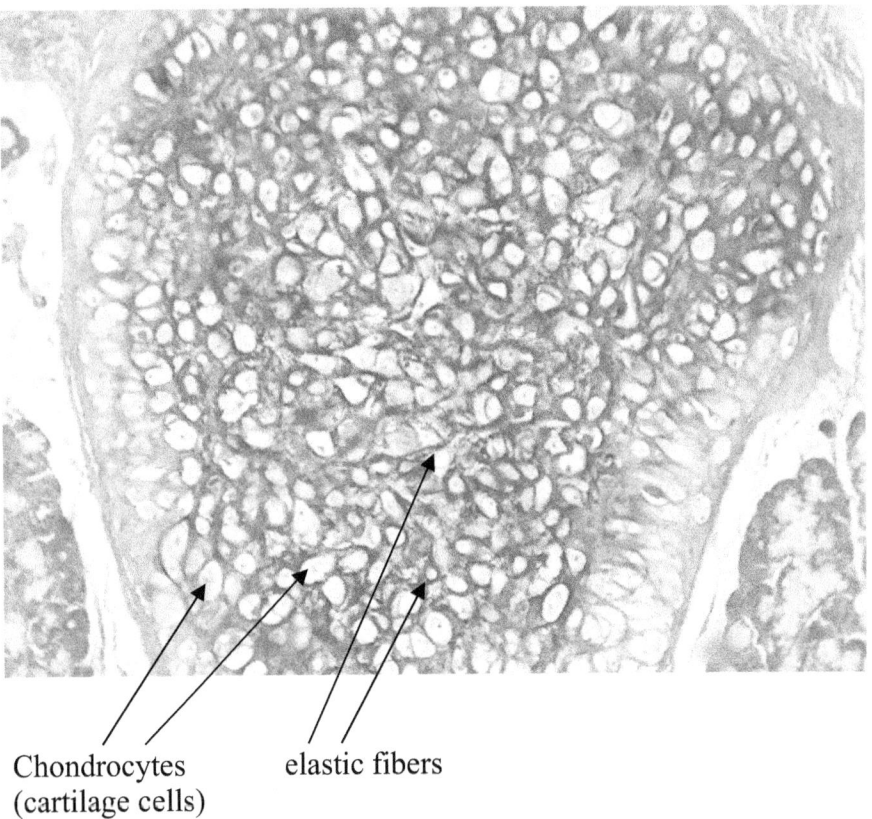

Chondrocytes   elastic fibers
(cartilage cells)

Elastic Cartilage at 100X

Elastic cartilage is much more flexible than the other cartilage types. This tissue can be found in abundance in our ears and epiglottis.

ELASTIC CARTILAGE

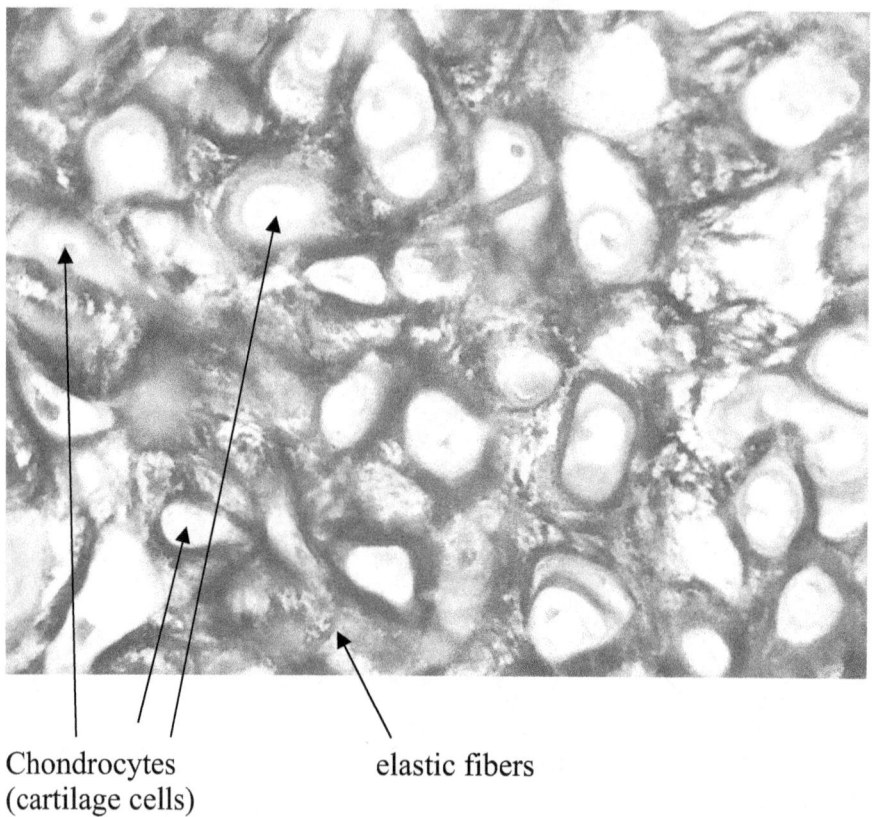

Chondrocytes (cartilage cells)   elastic fibers

Elastic cartilage at 400X

Chondrocytes are living cartilage cells.

Elastic cartilage is much more flexible than the other cartilage types. This tissue can be found in abundance in our ears and epiglottis.

EPIDIDYMIS

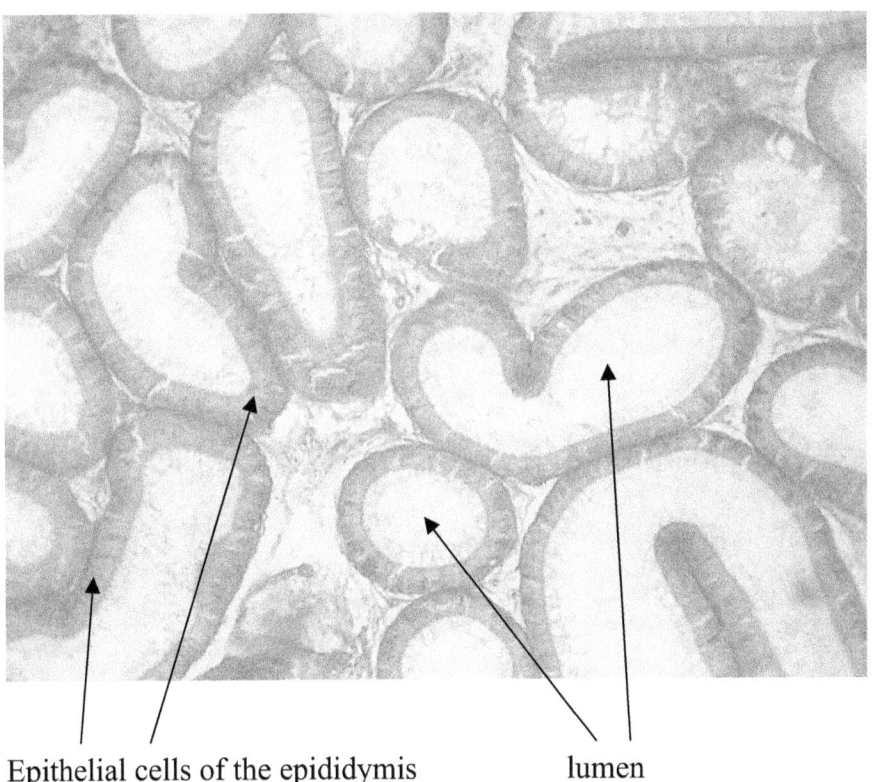

Epithelial cells of the epididymis   lumen

Epididymis at 100X

The epididymis is where sperm cells finish maturation.

EPIDIDYMIS

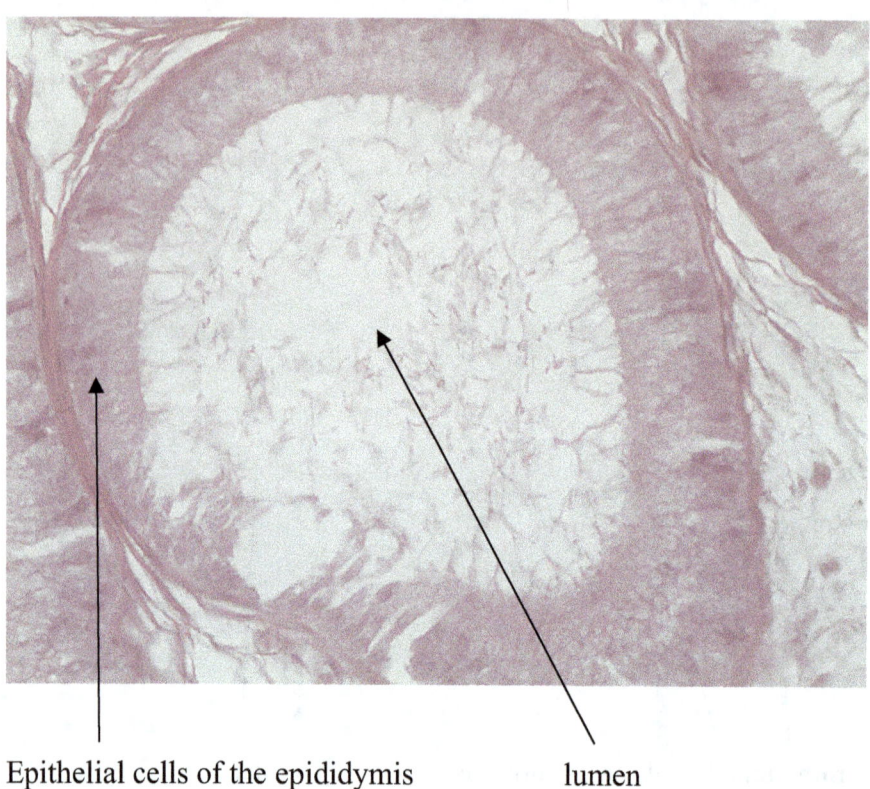

Epithelial cells of the epididymis   lumen

Epididymis at 400X

ESOPHAGUS

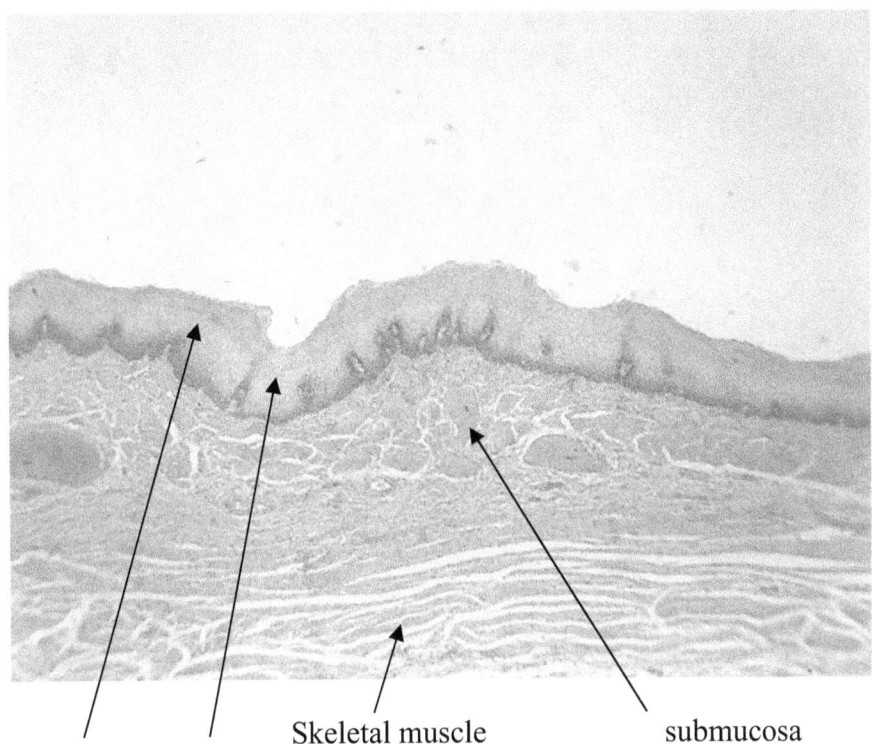

Stratified squamous layer of the mucosa (many flat layers) — Skeletal muscle — submucosa

Esophagus at 40X

The esophagus is a hollow muscular tube leading from the pharynx to the stomach.

The inner layer of the esophagus is stratified squamous epithelial tissue because a thick layer is needed for protection against abrasion and other potential damage.

ESOPHAGUS

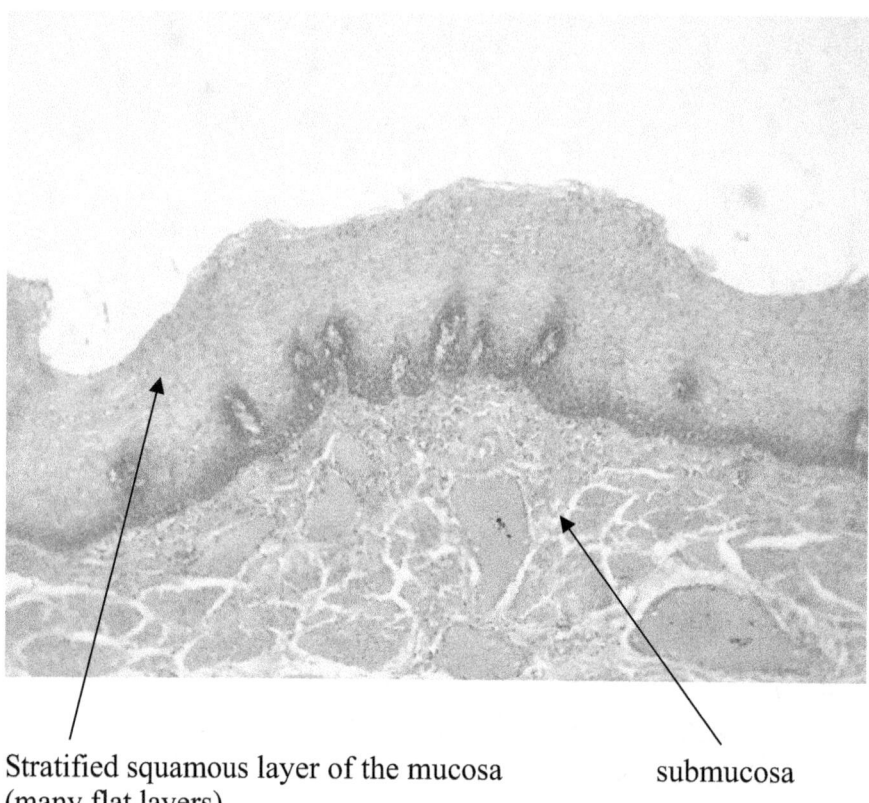

Stratified squamous layer of the mucosa submucosa
(many flat layers)

Esophagus at 100X

Where the esophagus passes through the diaphragm muscle there is a passageway called the esophageal hiatus. Sometimes a portion of the stomach may make its way into this opening and become constricted. This could cut off the oxygen supply to the tissue. A hiatal hernia is the passing of the stomach into this region.

ESOPHAGUS

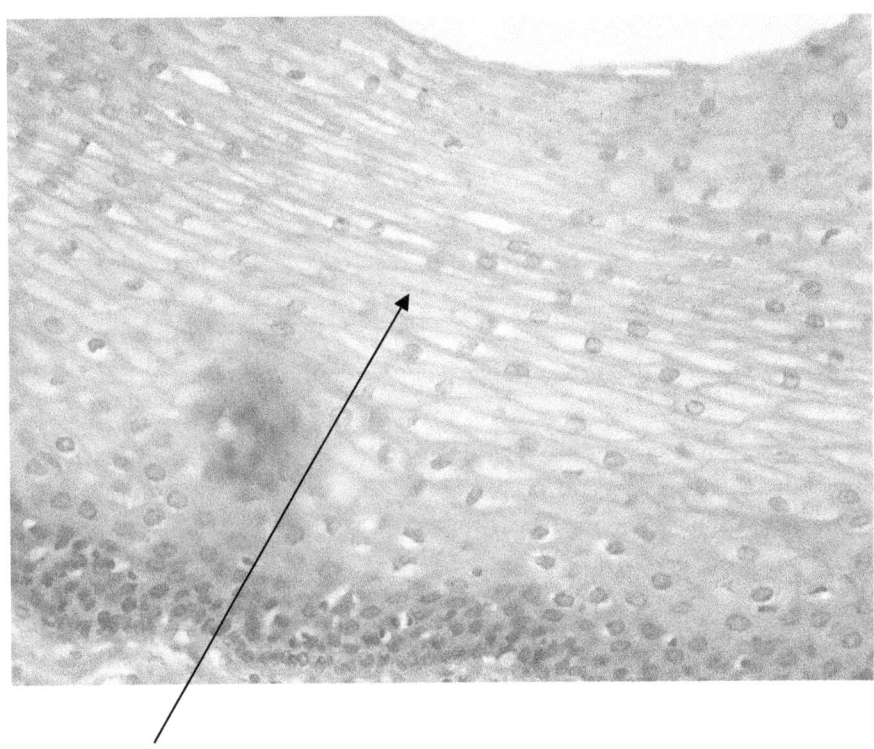

Stratified squamous layer of the mucosa
(many flat layers)

Esophagus at 400X

ESOPHAGEAL CARDIAC JUNCTION

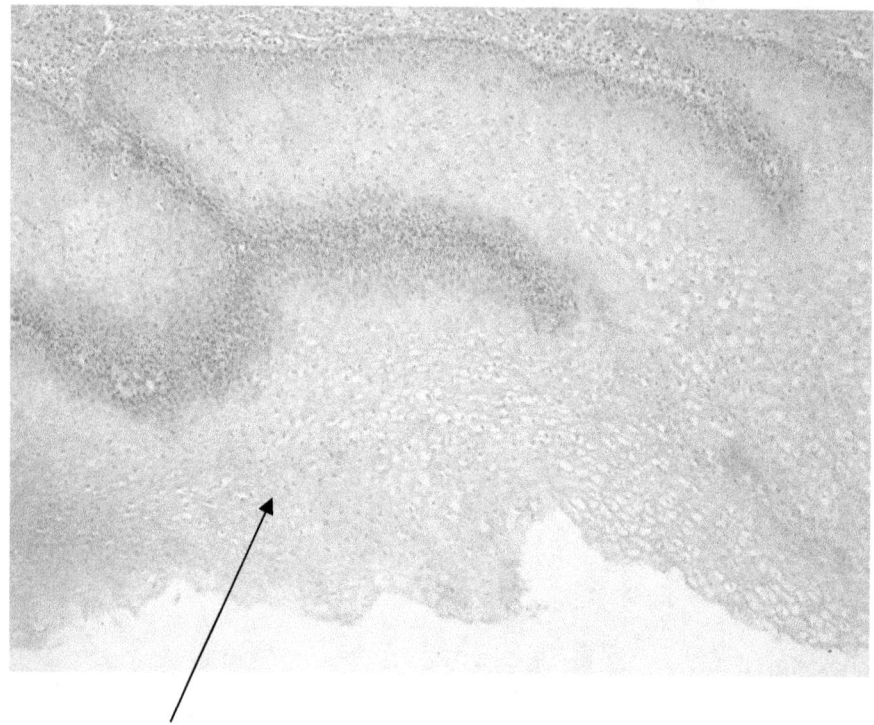

Stratified squamous layer
(many flat layers)

Esophageal cardiac junction at 100X

ESOPHAGEAL CARDIAC JUNCTION

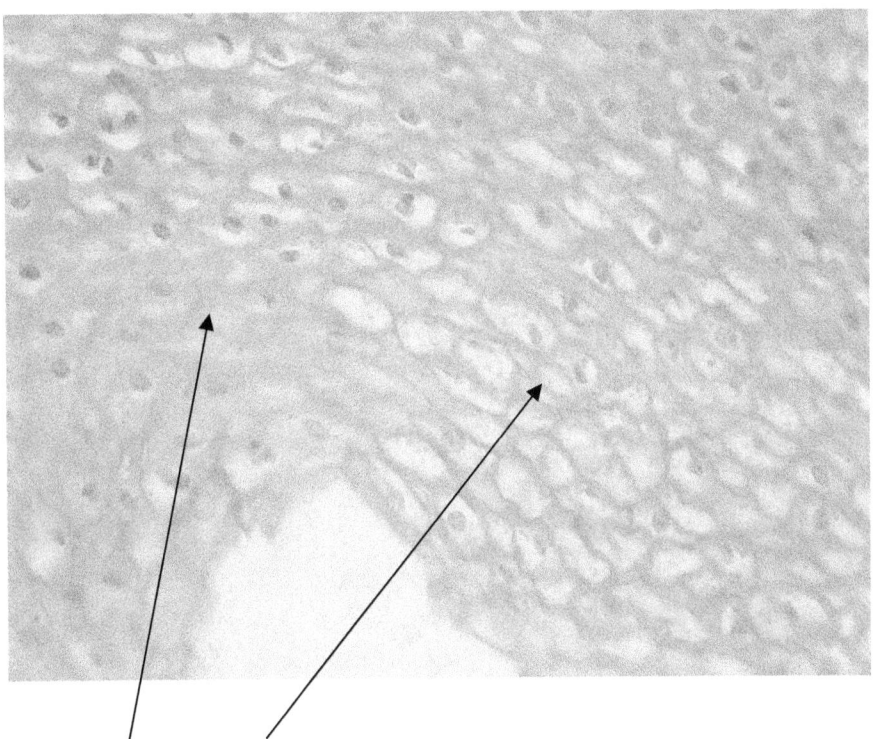

Stratified squamous layer
(many flat layers)

Esophageal cardiac junction at 400X

FALLOPIAN TUBE (ISTHMUS)

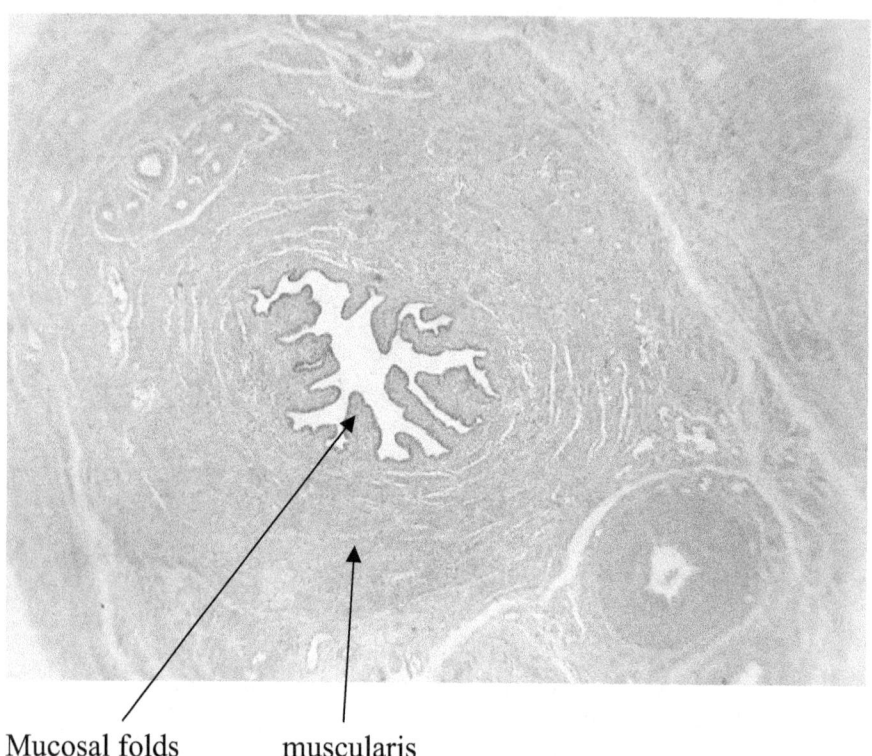

Mucosal folds   muscularis

Fallopian tube at 40X

The fallopian tubes are also called the uterine tubes or ovarian tubes. These tubes connect the ovaries to the uterus and are responsible for moving an oocyte or developing embryo if fertilization were to take place. The inside of the fallopian tubes are lined with cilia. These cilia will move the oocyte or embryo over the cell surface towards the uterus.

FALLOPIAN TUBE (ISTHMUS)

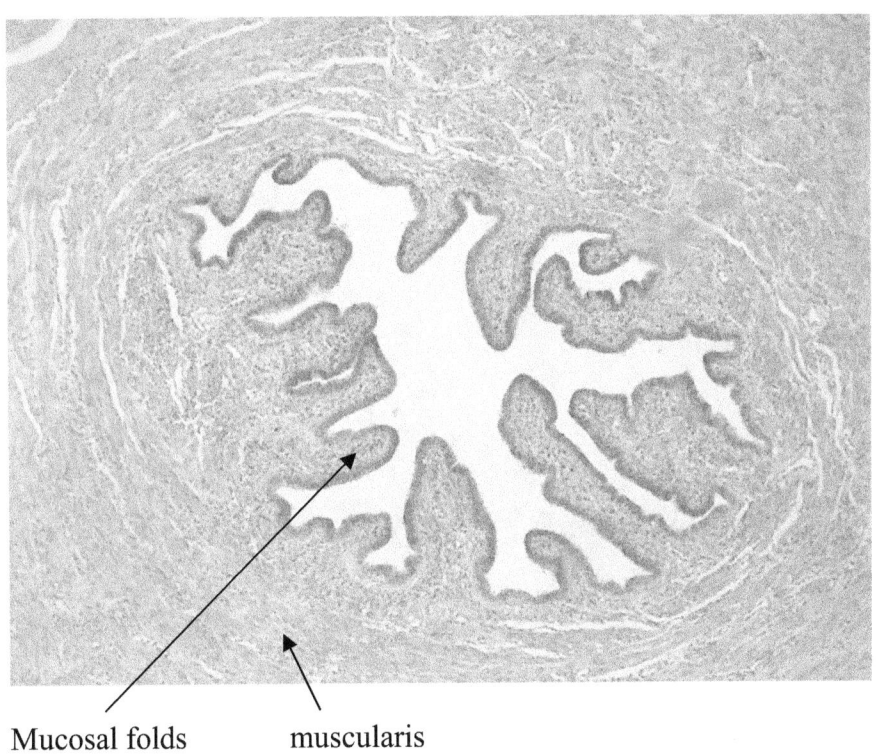

Mucosal folds   muscularis

Fallopian tube at 100X

FALLOPIAN TUBE (ISTHMUS)

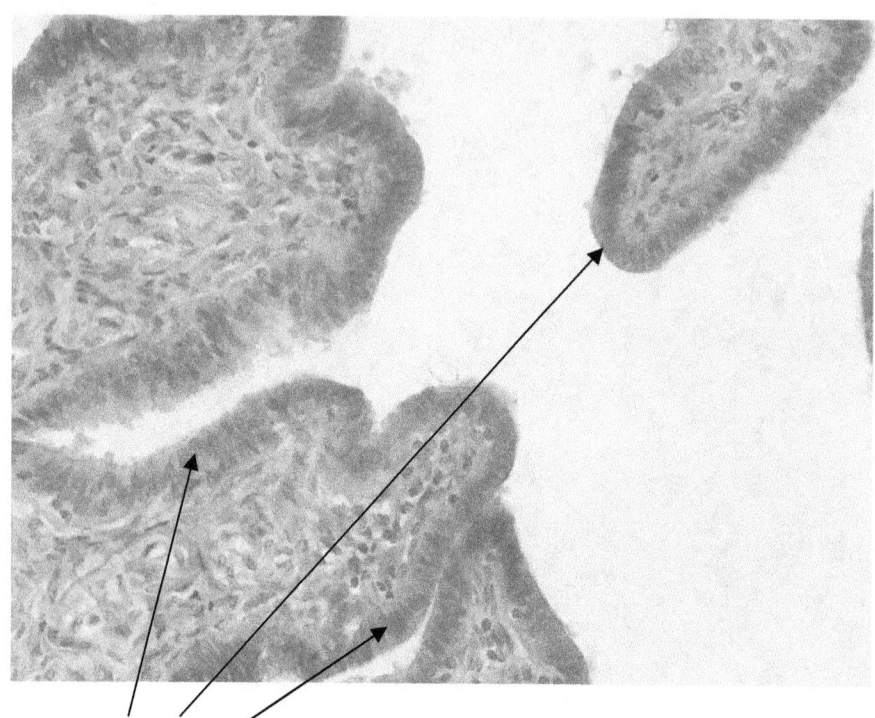

Simple columnar cells with cilia
(1 tall, thin layer)

Fallopian tube at 400X

GALLBLADDER

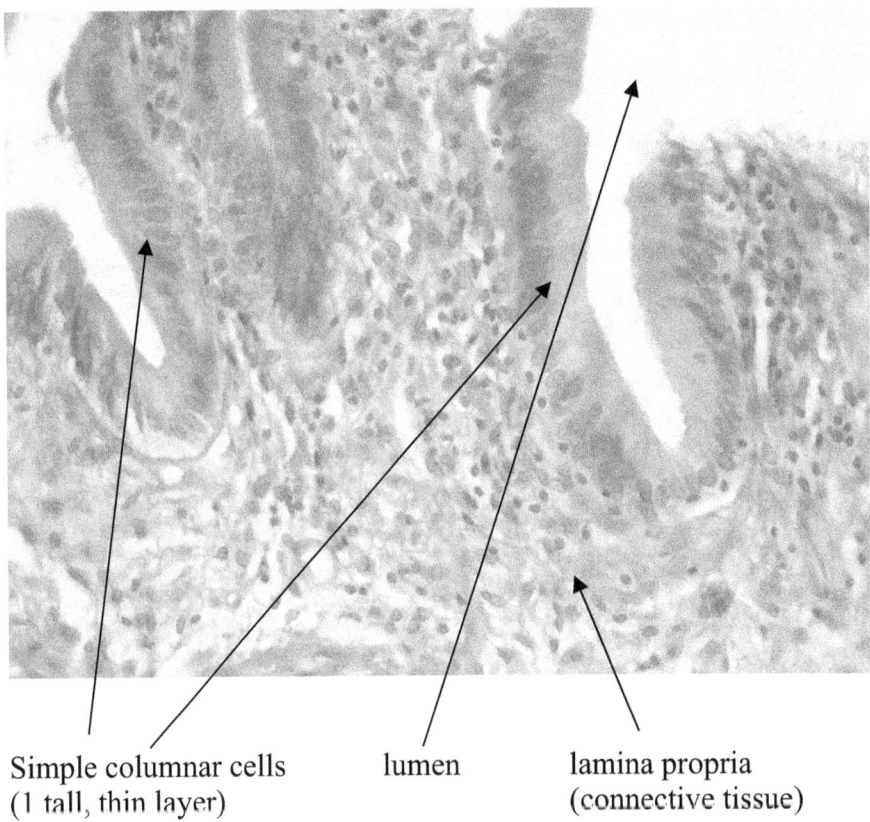

Simple columnar cells   lumen   lamina propria
(1 tall, thin layer)   (connective tissue)

Gallbladder at 400X

The gallbladder is a hollow muscular organ, which only stores bile. The gallbladder doesn't produce anything.

GOBLET CELLS

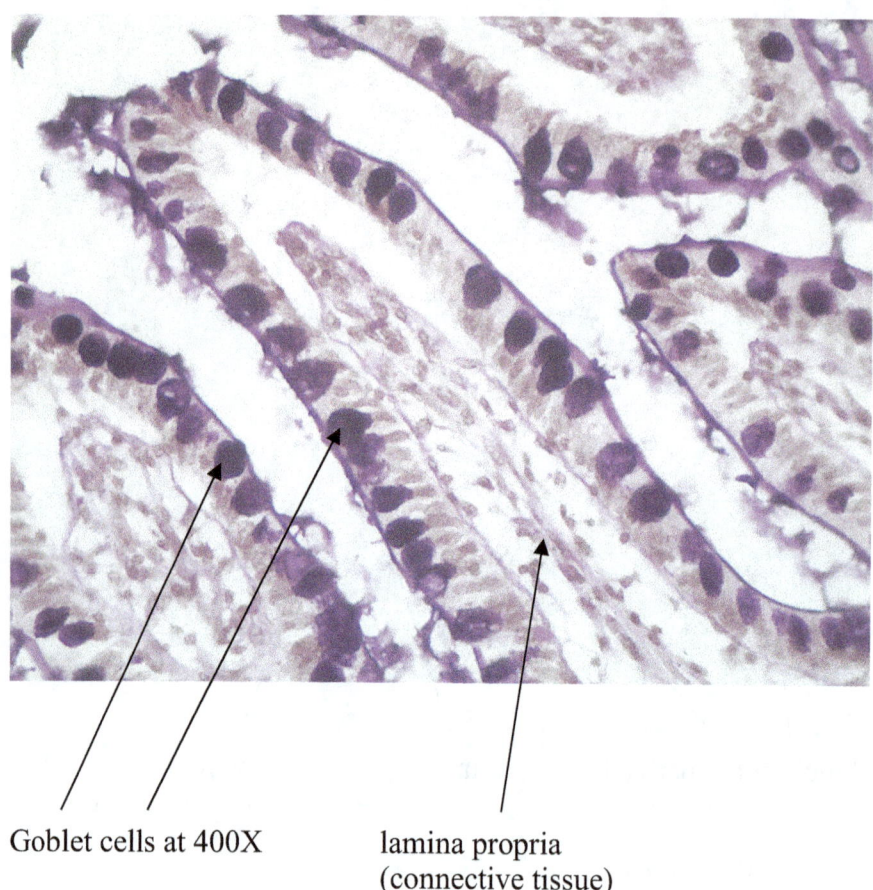

Goblet cells at 400X

lamina propria
(connective tissue)

Goblet cells are mucous producing cells of the body.

GOBLET CELLS IN THE ILEUM

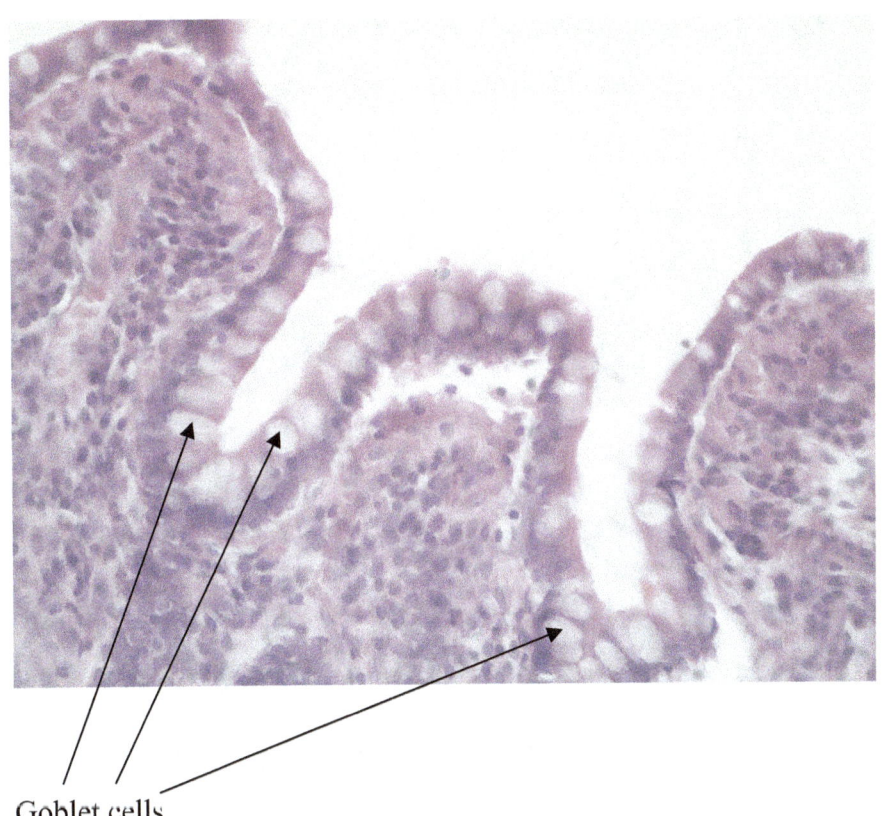

Goblet cells

Goblet cells in the ileum at 400X

HYPOPHYSIS (Pituitary gland)

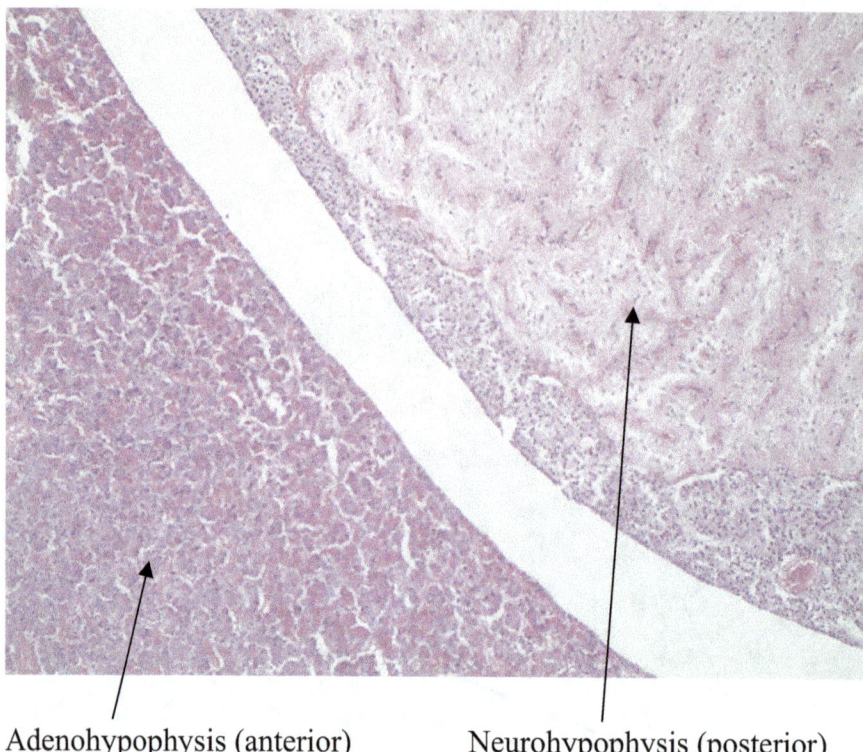

Adenohypophysis (anterior)   Neurohypophysis (posterior)

Hypophysis at 100X

Neurohypophysis – this is the rear (posterior) half of the pituitary gland and is the site where ADH (antidiuretic hormone) and oxytocin are released.

Adenohypophysis – this is the front (anterior) half of the pituitary gland and releases lipotropins, beta endorphins, growth hormone, thyroid stimulating hormone, adrenocorticotropic hormone, luteinizing hormone, follicle stimulating hormone, melanocyte stimulating hormone and prolactin.

HYPOPHYSIS (Pituitary gland)

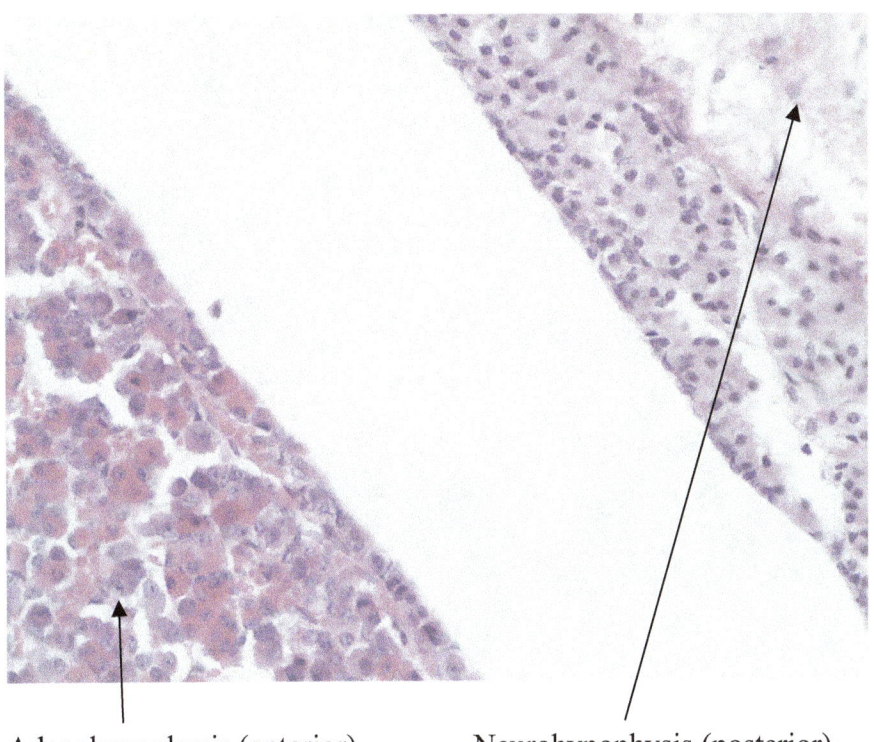

Adenohypophysis (anterior)   Neurohypophysis (posterior)

Hypophysis at 400X

The adenohypophysis is connected to the hypothalamus by the hypothalamohypophysial portal system. A portal system will always be a direct connection between two areas. This portal system allows for precise hormone control between these two areas.

The neurohypophysis is connected to the hypothalamus by the hypothalamohypophysial tract system. This tract is a bundle of axons connecting the hypothalamus to the posterior pituitary.

INTESTINE

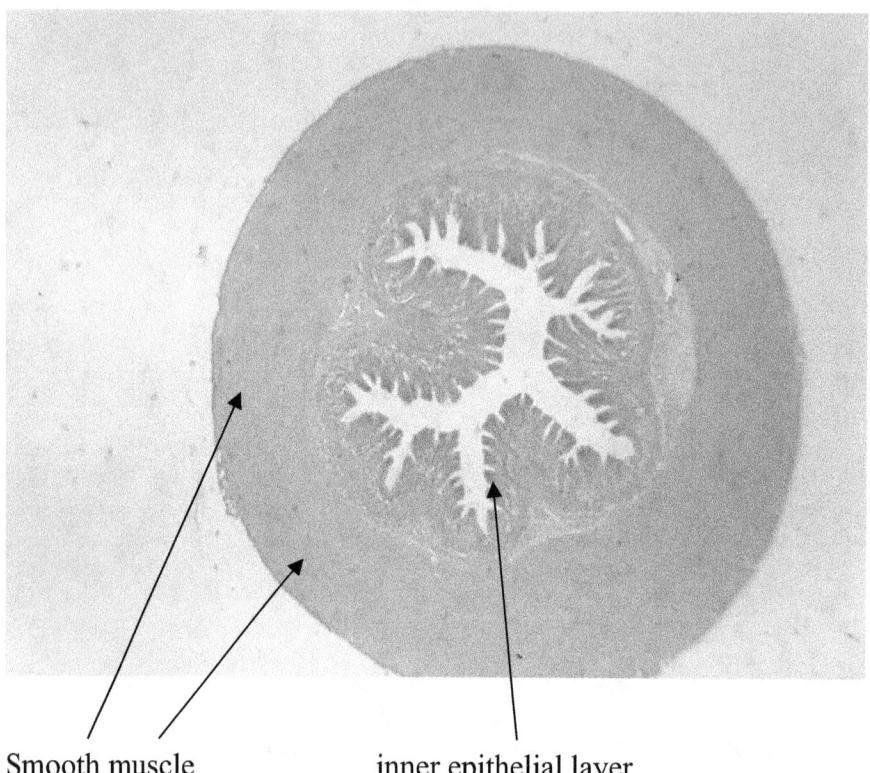

Smooth muscle   inner epithelial layer

Intestine at 40X

The intestines are made mostly of smooth muscle, with an inner epithelial tissue lining the lumen (hollow center). This muscle will move materials through the GI tract.

INTESTINE (SMOOTH MUSCLE)

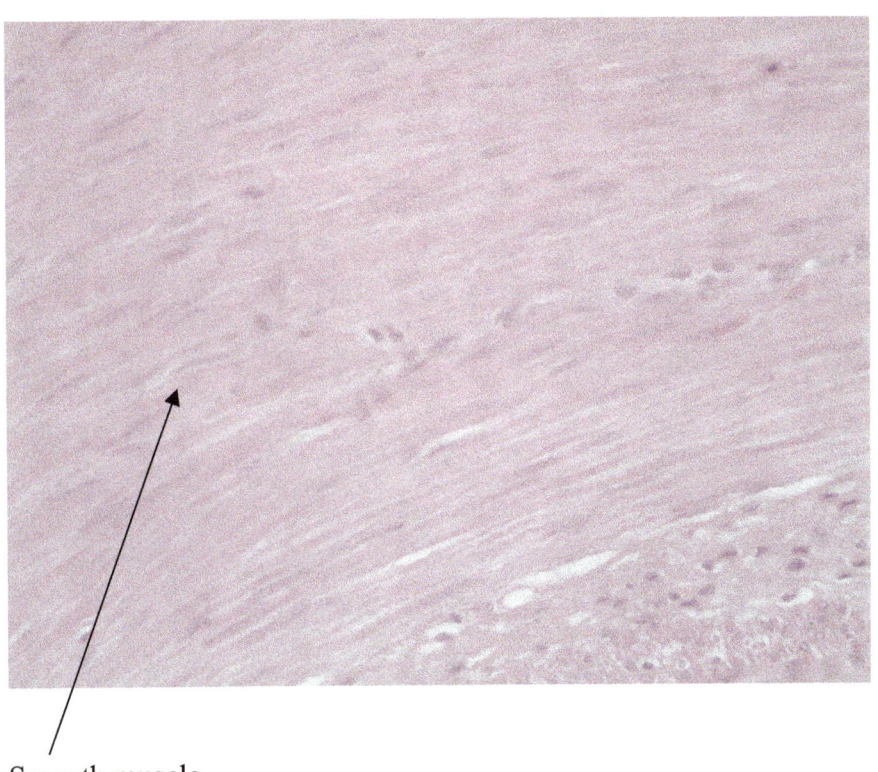

Smooth muscle

Intestine (smooth muscle) at 400X

INTESTINE

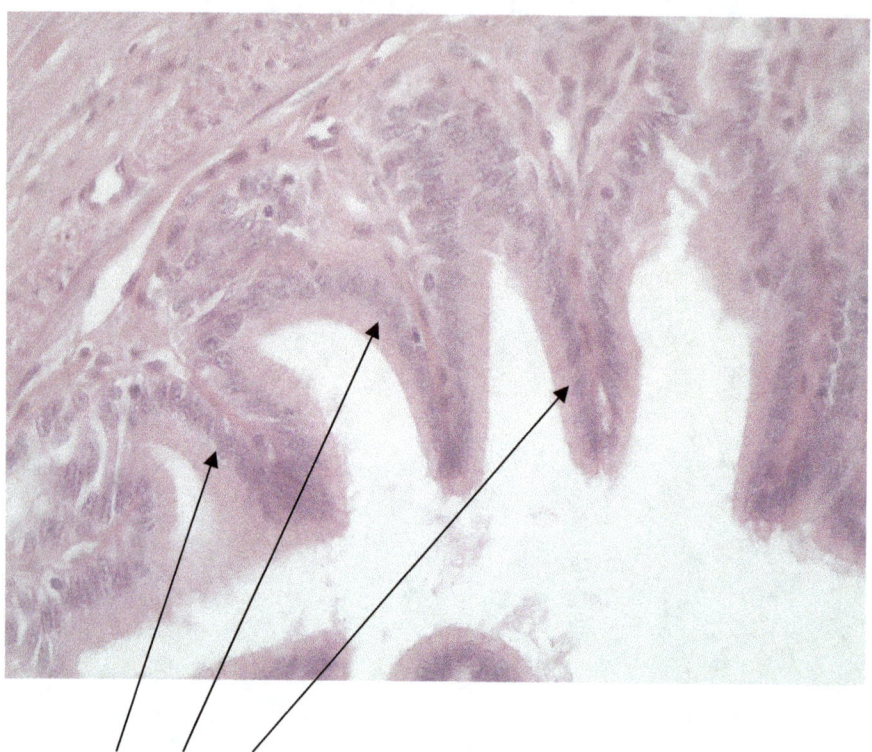

Simple columnar layer
(1 tall, thin layer)

Intestine at 400X

KIDNEYS

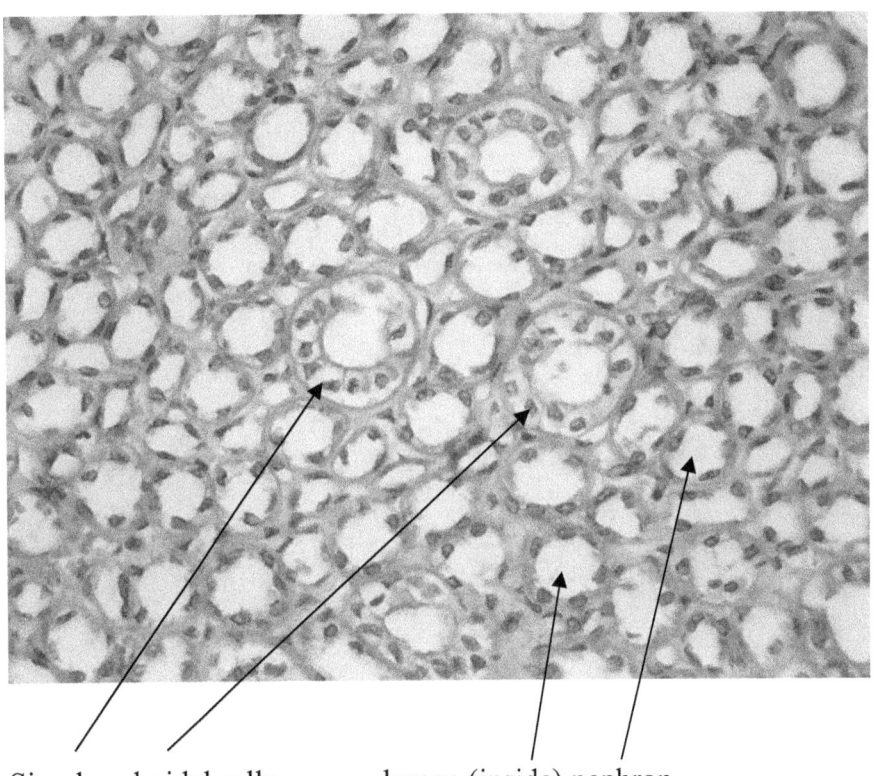

Simple cuboidal cells
(1 cube shaped layer)

lumen (inside) nephron

Nephrons (tubules)

Kidneys at 400X

The kidneys are filled with tube like structures called nephrons. In this picture you are seeing the inside of these tubes.

Each tube is made of one, cube shaped layer of epithelial cells. The cells are side by side, making the walls of the tubes.

KIDNEYS

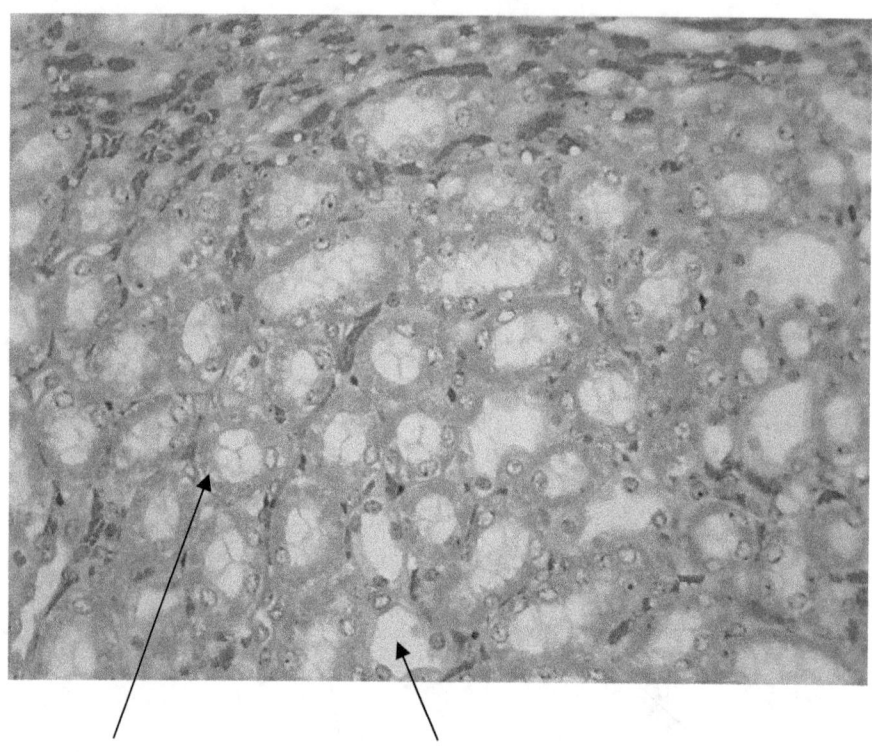

Simple cuboidal cells
(1 cube shaped layer)

lumen (inside) nephron

Kidneys at 400X

A nephron has many sections to it. Some of the larger sections are the Bowman's capsule, the proximal tubule, the loop of Henle and the distal tubule. In some areas of the nephrons the cells are cuboidal and in regions of the loop of Henle they are squamous.

LARGE INTESTINE

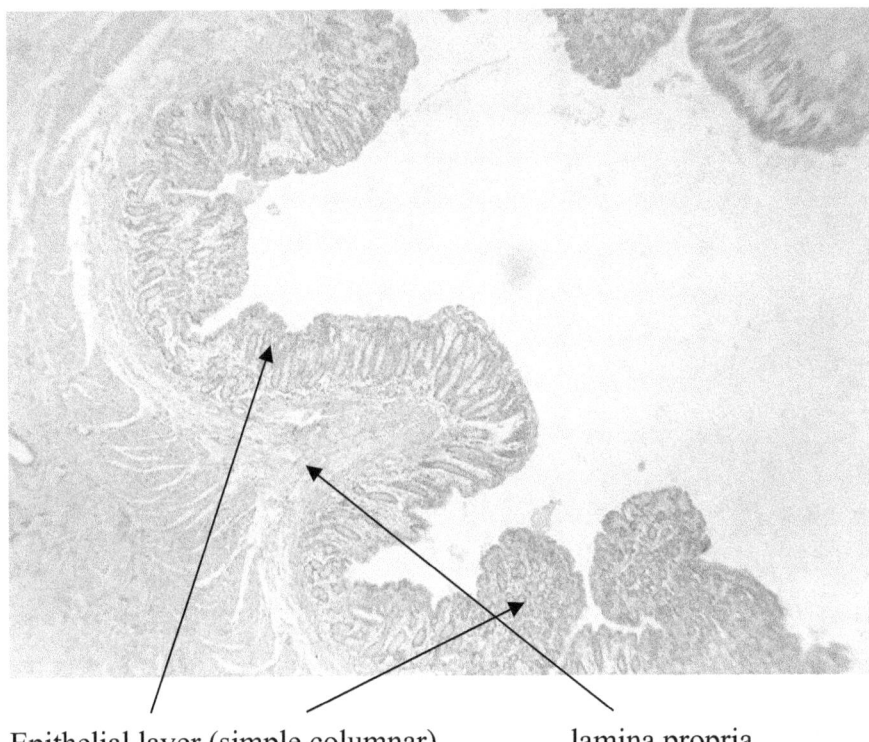

Epithelial layer (simple columnar)   lamina propria
                                       (connective tissue)

Large intestine at 40X

In the large intestine most of the remaining water is reabsorbed back into the body. The contractions of the smooth muscle in this area are referred to as mass movements.

The large intestine contains many helpful microorganisms, and we enjoy a nice symbiotic relationship with them. One of the helpful materials bacteria in the large intestine make for us is vitamin K. The actions of bacteria in the large intestine produce a gas we call flatus.

LARGE INTESTINE

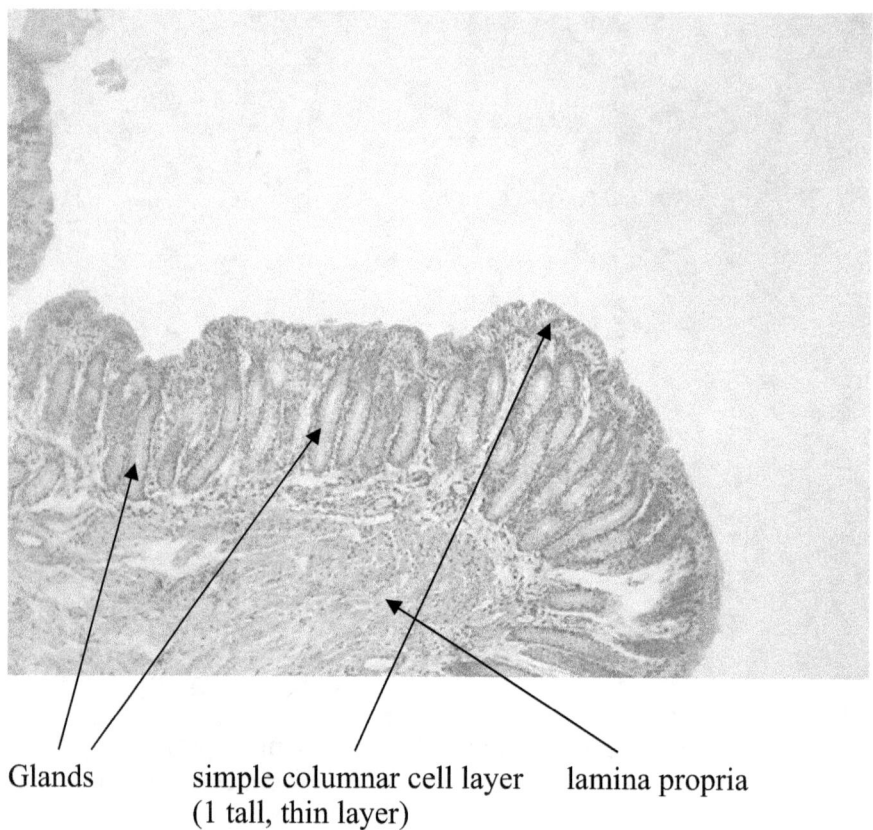

Glands   simple columnar cell layer   lamina propria
           (1 tall, thin layer)

Large intestine at 100X

Along the large intestine are many small segments which look like pouches. These pouches are called haustra. Haustra can't be seen in a slide, they are much too large.

LARGE INTESTINE

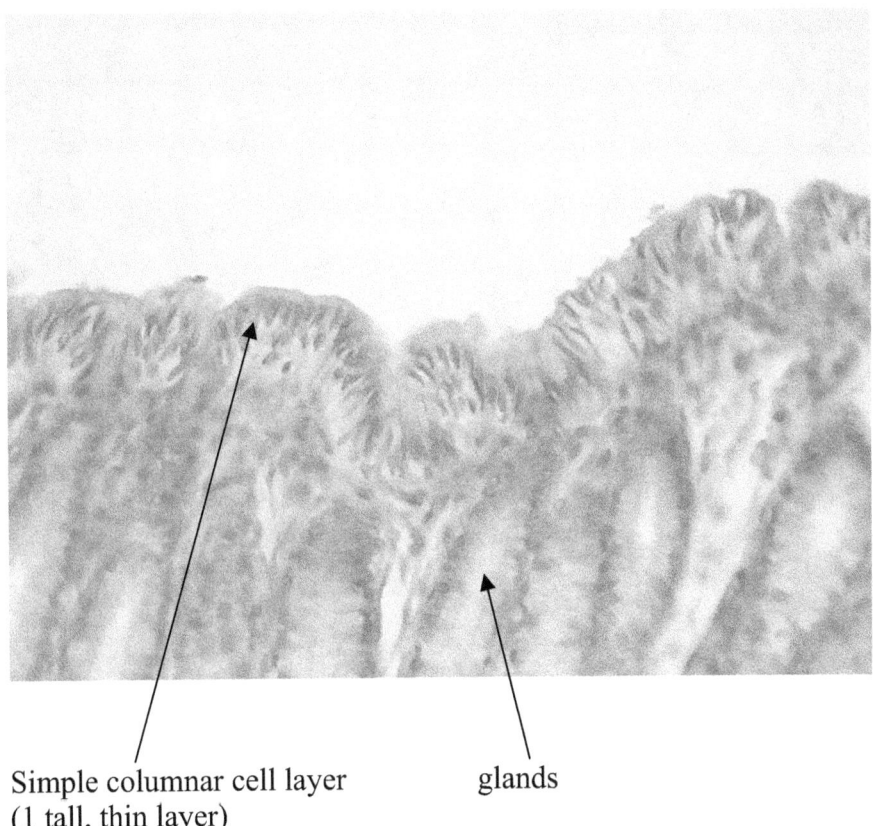

Simple columnar cell layer
(1 tall, thin layer)

glands

Large intestine at 400X

The tall thin layer of epithelial tissue comes into focus at 400X.

The large intestine has many fatty deposits on its superficial surface. These deposits are called epiploic appendages.

As the cells of the large intestine reabsorb most of the remaining water, the remaining material will leave the body as what we call feces.

LIVER

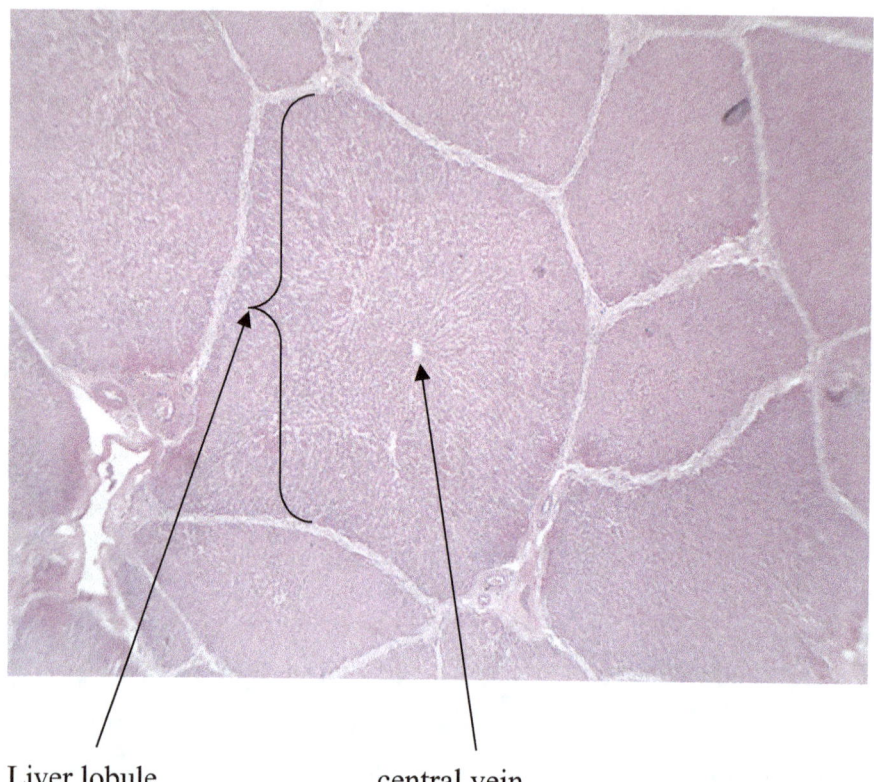

Liver lobule   central vein

Liver at 40X

The liver has six major functions: detoxification, bile production, storage, synthesizing nutrients, synthesizing plasma proteins and phagocytizing old red blood cells. The liver is a very large internal organ and takes up much of the space in the upper right quadrant of the abdominal cavity.

LIVER

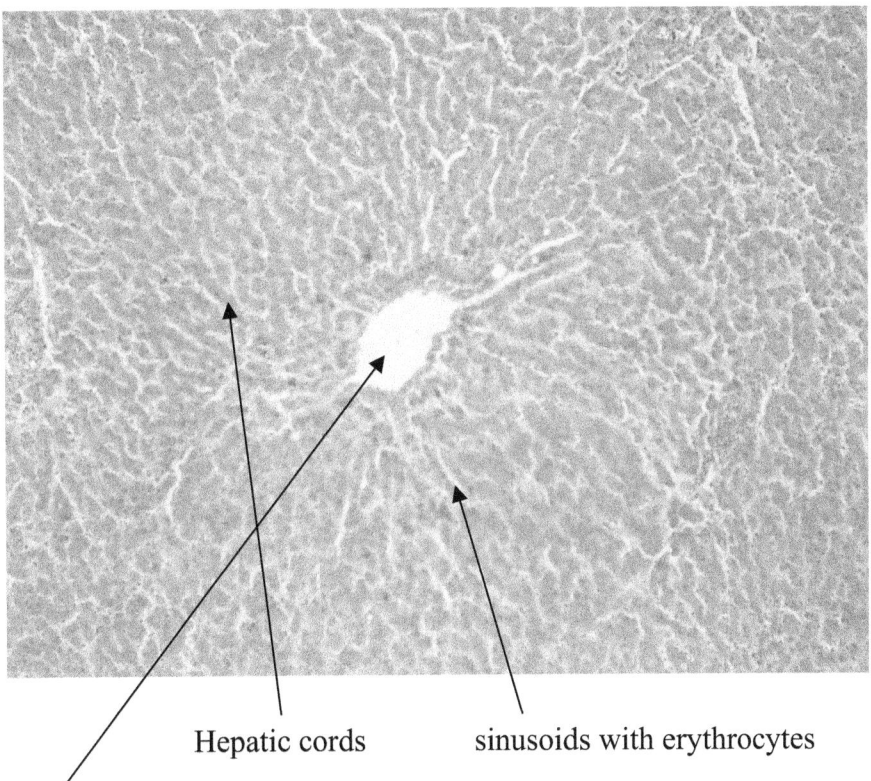

Hepatic cords   sinusoids with erythrocytes

Central vein surrounded by hepatic cords made up of hepatocytes.

One liver lobule shown in picture.

Liver at 40X

The liver is divided into many lobules and each lobule is made of many hepatic cords. Each hepatic cord radiates out from the center of the lobule like spokes on a bicycle tire. Each cord is made of many liver cells called hepatocytes.

LIVER

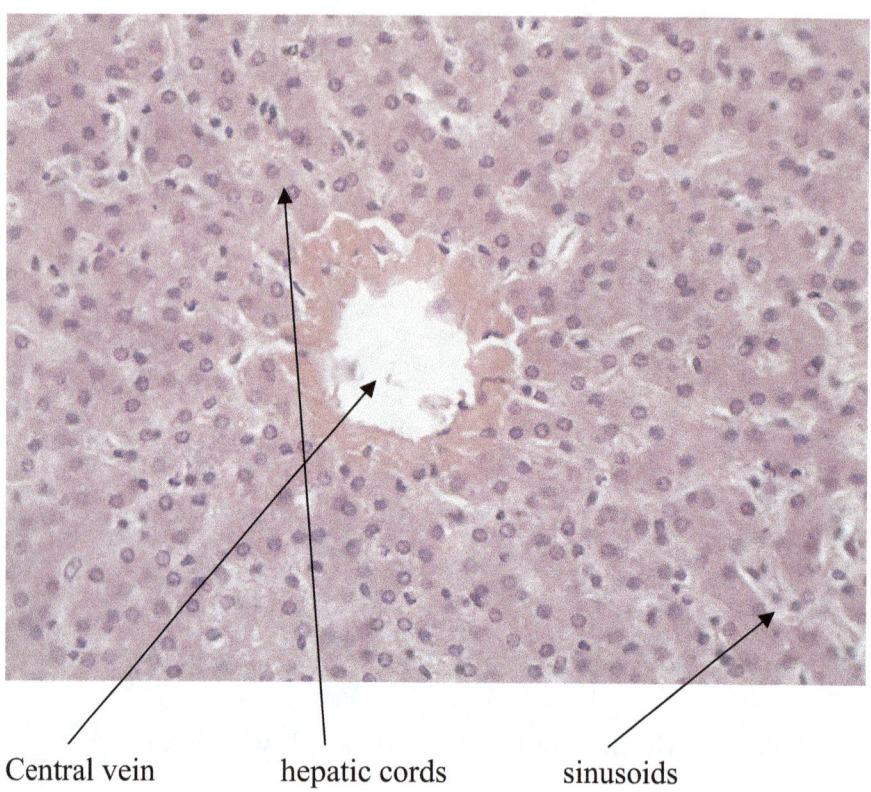

Central vein   hepatic cords   sinusoids

Central vein surrounded by hepatocytes (liver cells)

Liver at 100X

LIVER

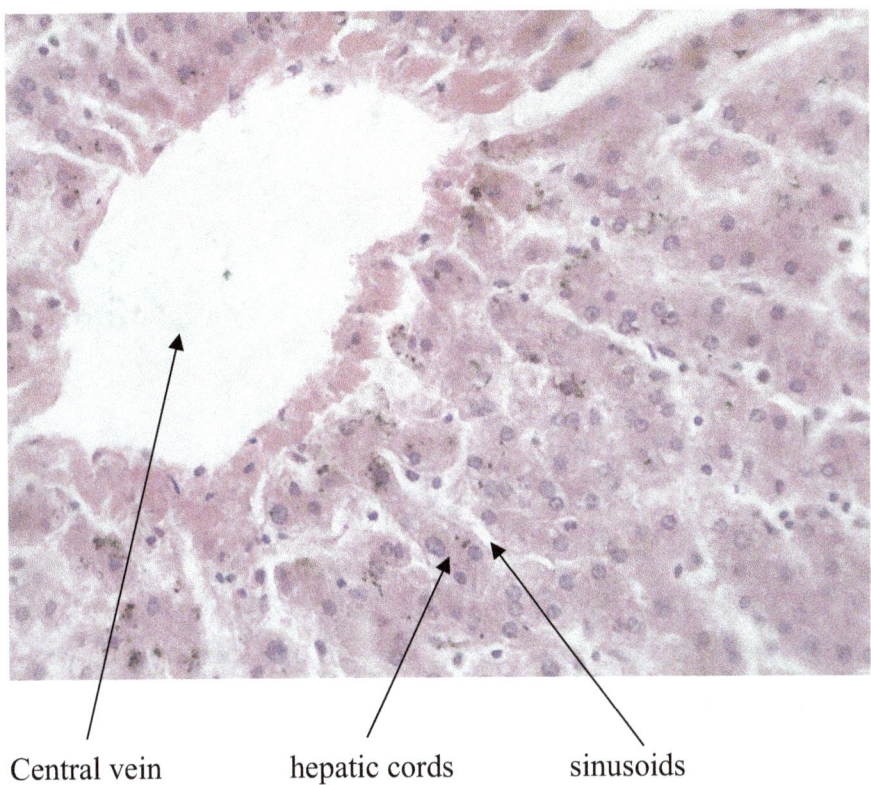

Central vein   hepatic cords   sinusoids

Central vein surrounded by hepatocytes (liver cells)

Liver at 400X

LOOSE CONNECTIVE TISSUE

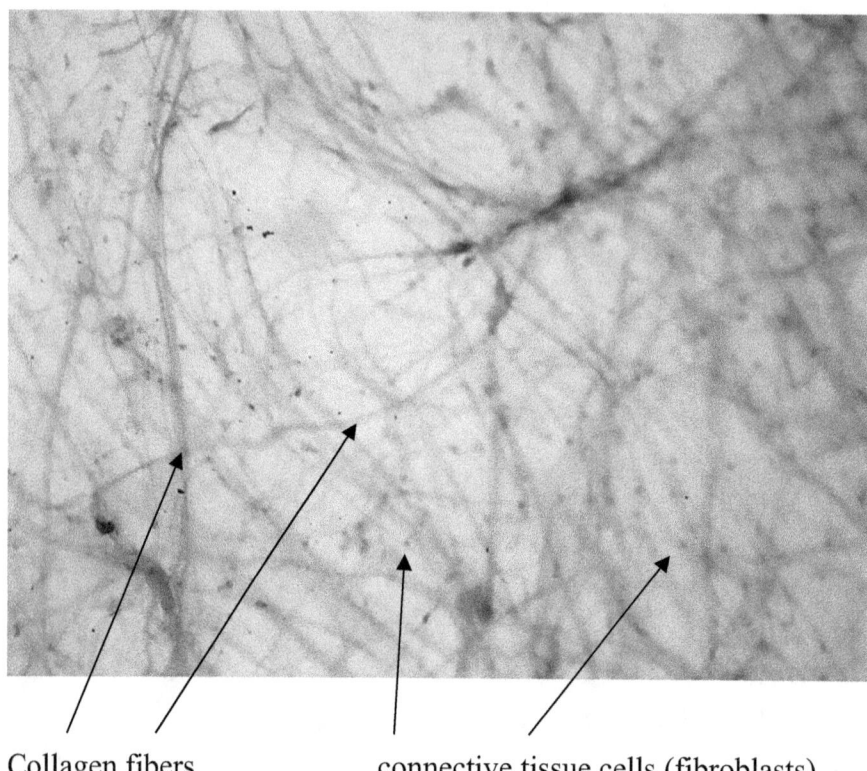

Collagen fibers connective tissue cells (fibroblasts)

Loose connective tissue at 100X

Loose connective tissue gets its name because the fibers have lots of space in between them. There are 3 fibers commonly found in connective tissue, they are collagen, elastic and reticular.

Loose connective tissue is also called areolar tissue.

LOOSE CONNECTIVE TISSUE

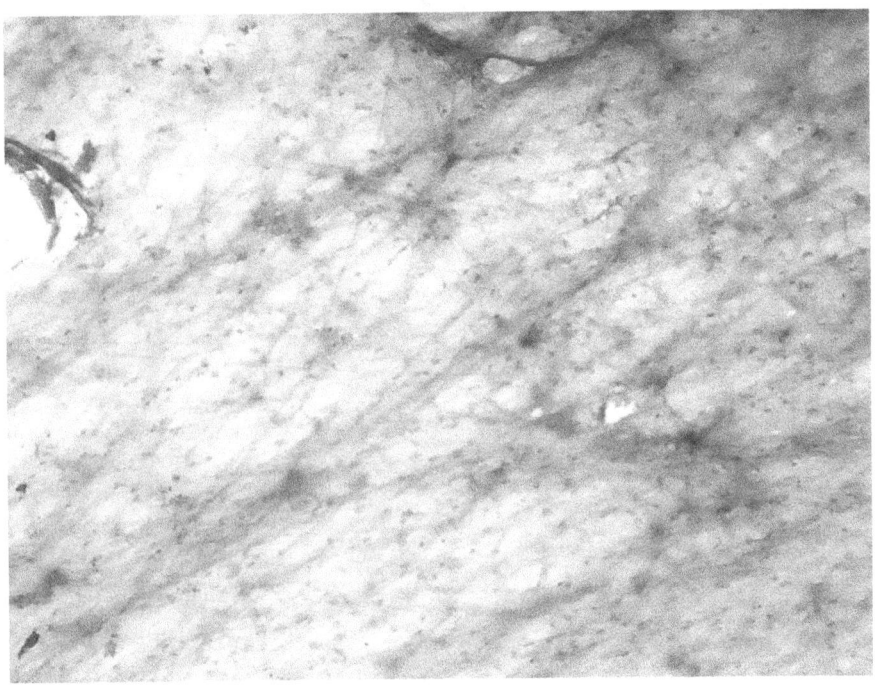

Loose connective tissue at 100X

Notice the large amount of space in between all of the fibers and cells.

LOOSE CONNECTIVE TISSUE

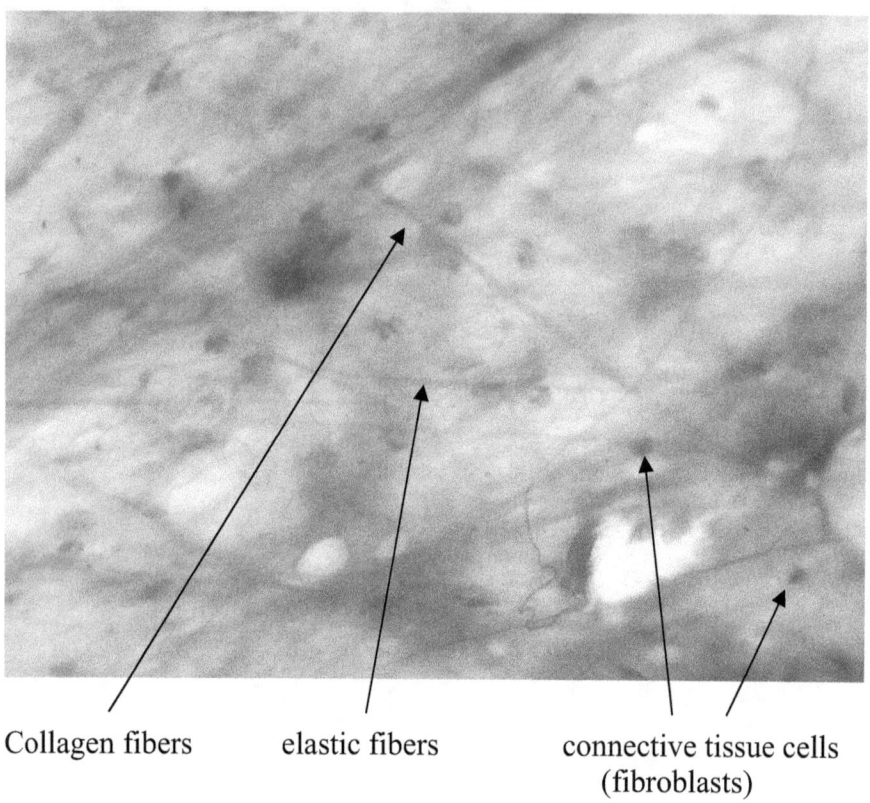

Collagen fibers   elastic fibers   connective tissue cells
                                     (fibroblasts)

Loose connective tissue at 400X

LUNG

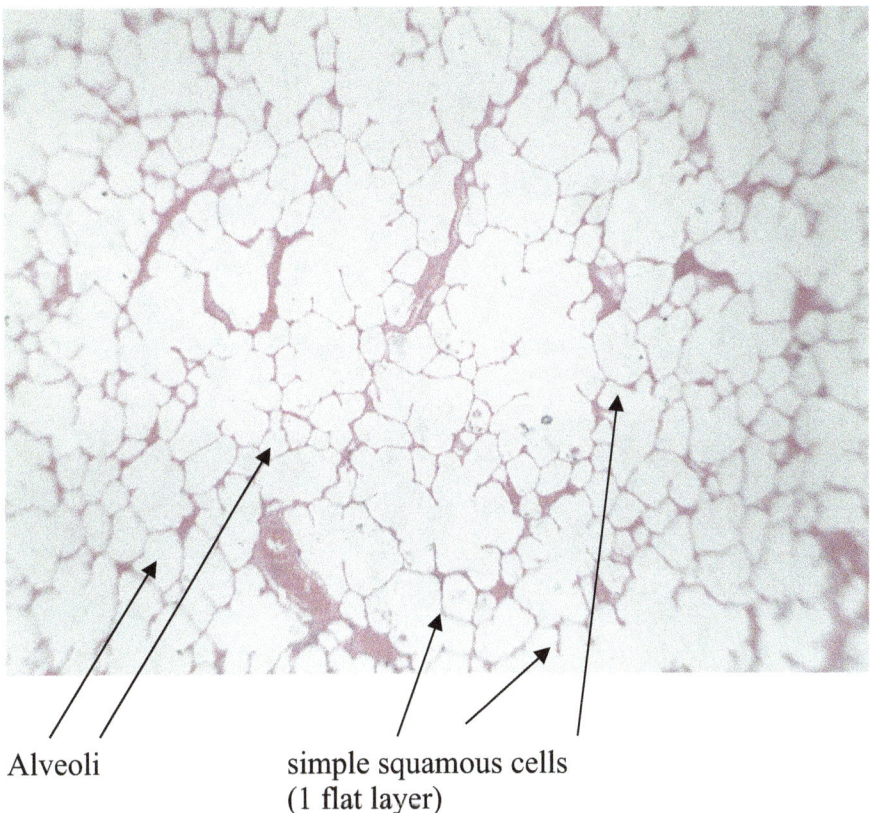

Alveoli   simple squamous cells
(1 flat layer)

Lung at 40X

The lungs are filled with millions of tiny air sacs called alveoli. The alveoli can be seen in the picture above. Each alveoli is surrounded by two types of epithelial cells called pneumocytes. Most of the epithelial cells are simple squamous and are there for gas exchange. One simple layer of cells is as thin as it gets, and thin layers are good for swapping materials. The remaining cells are simple cuboidal and are there to produce surfactant. Surfactant decreases the attraction of water molecules. Without the surfactant the water would pull the alveolar walls together every time we exhaled, and our lungs would collapse.

LUNG

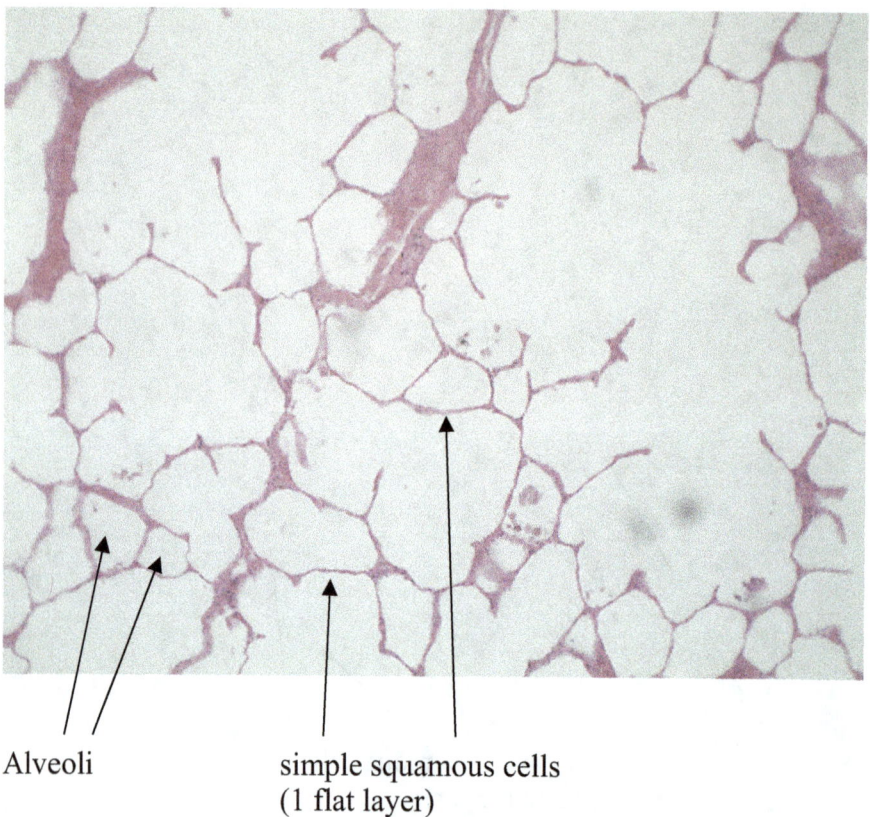

Alveoli simple squamous cells
(1 flat layer)

Lung at 100X

The lungs are filled with millions of tiny air sacs called alveoli. The alveoli can be seen in the picture above. Each alveoli is surrounded by two types of epithelial cells called pneumocytes. Most of the epithelial cells are simple squamous and are there for gas exchange. One simple layer of cells is as thin as it gets, and thin layers are good for swapping materials. The remaining cells are simple cuboidal and are there to produce surfactant. Surfactant decreases the attraction of water molecules. Without the surfactant the water would pull the alveolar walls together every time we exhaled, and our lungs would collapse.

LUNG

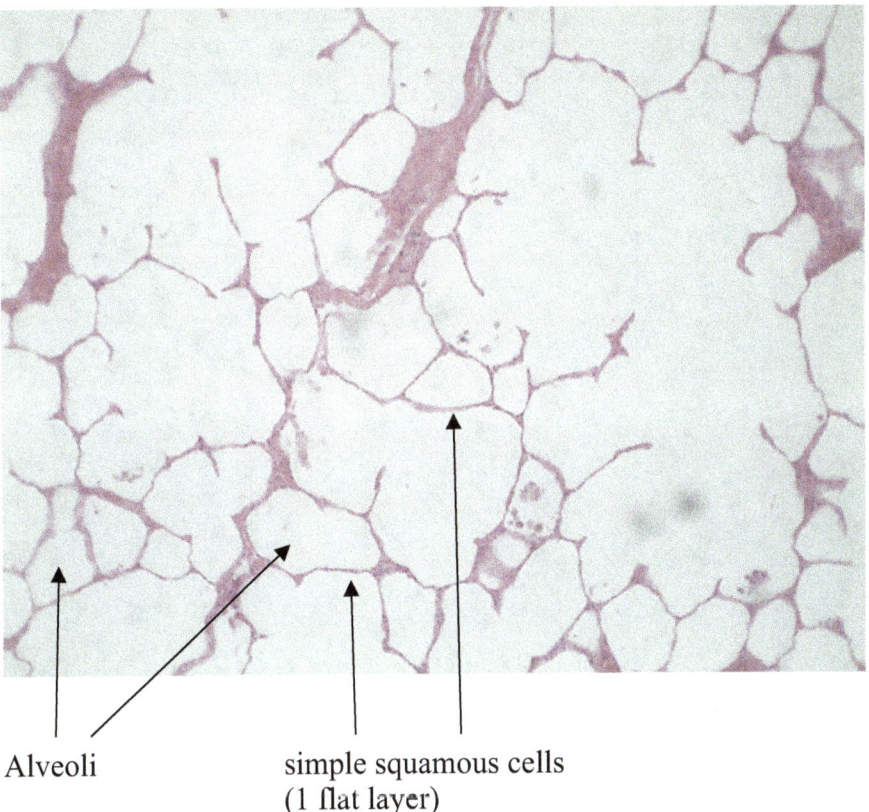

Alveoli — simple squamous cells (1 flat layer)

Lung at 100X

The lungs are filled with millions of tiny air sacs called alveoli. The alveoli can be seen in the picture above. Each alveoli is surrounded by two types of epithelial cells called pneumocytes. Most of the epithelial cells are simple squamous and are there for gas exchange. One simple layer of cells is as thin as it gets, and thin layers are good for swapping materials. The remaining cells are simple cuboidal and are there to produce surfactant. Surfactant decreases the attraction of water molecules. Without the surfactant the water would pull the alveolar walls together every time we exhaled, and our lungs would collapse.

LUNG WITH CARBON

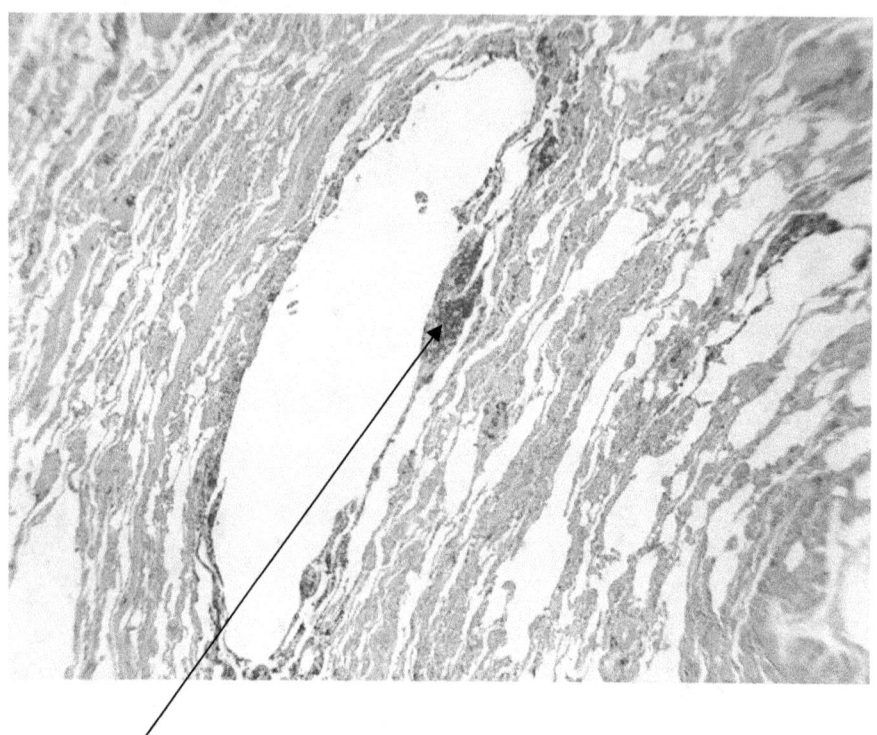

Carbon in lungs

Lung with carbon at 40X

LUNG WITH CARBON

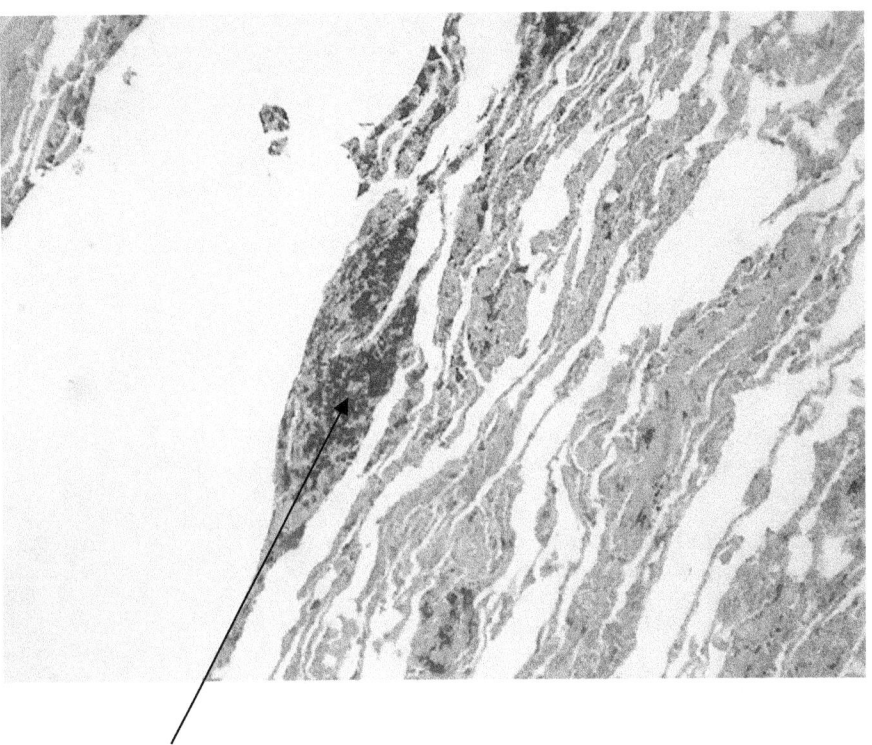

Carbon in lungs

Lung with carbon at 100X

LYMPH NODE

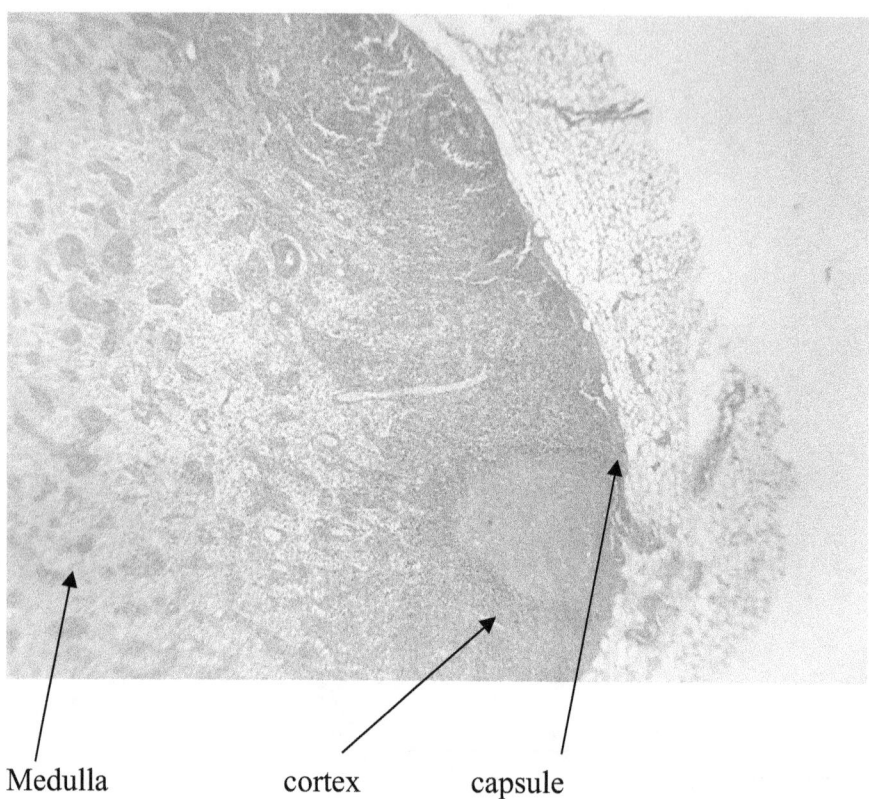

Medulla   cortex   capsule

Lymph node at 40X

A lymph node is surrounded by a connective tissue layer called a capsule. The inside of the node is separated into an outer cortex and an inner medulla. Reticular fibers form the supporting framework for all the lymphocytes.

Lymph nodes filter lymph (fluids) returning from many tissues of the body.

LYMPH NODE

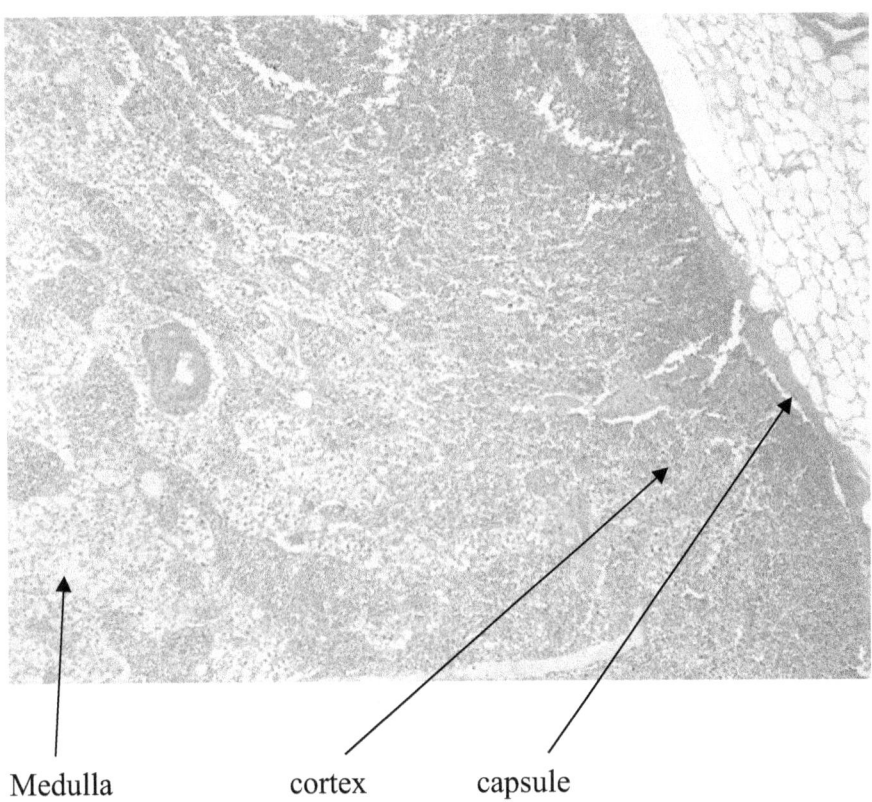

Medulla   cortex   capsule

Lymph node at 100X

A lymph node is surrounded by a connective tissue layer called a capsule. The inside of the node is separated into an outer cortex and an inner medulla. Reticular fibers form the supporting framework for all the lymphocytes.

Lymph nodes filter lymph (fluids) returning from many tissues of the body.

LYMPH NODE

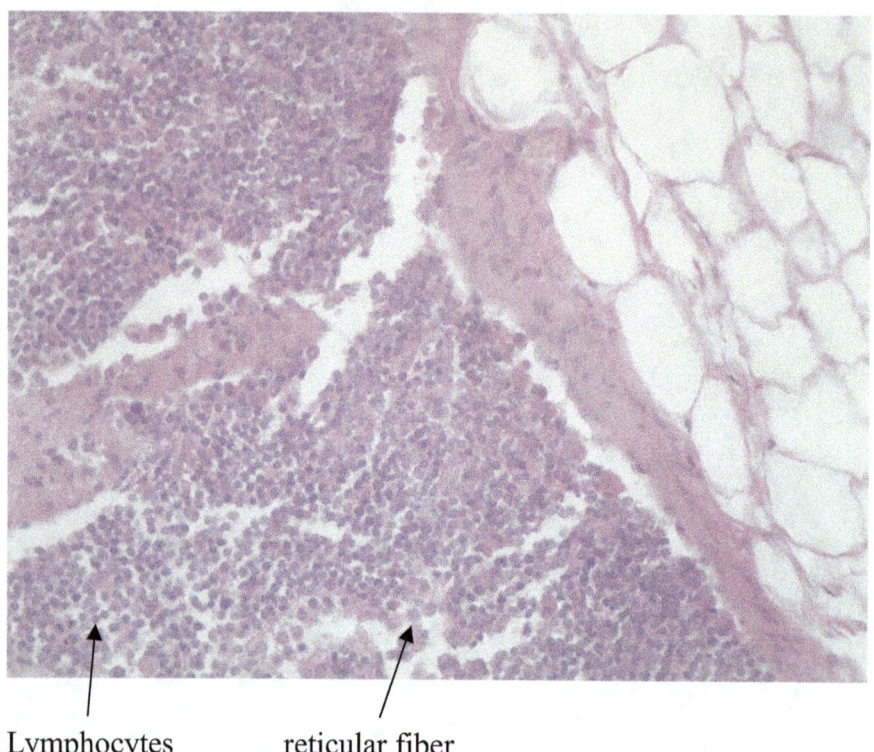

Lymphocytes   reticular fiber

Lymph node at 400X

A lymph node is surrounded by a connective tissue layer called a capsule. The inside of the node is separated into an outer cortex and an inner medulla. Reticular fibers form the supporting framework for all the lymphocytes.

Lymph nodes filter lymph (fluids) returning from many tissues of the body.

MAMMARY GLANDS

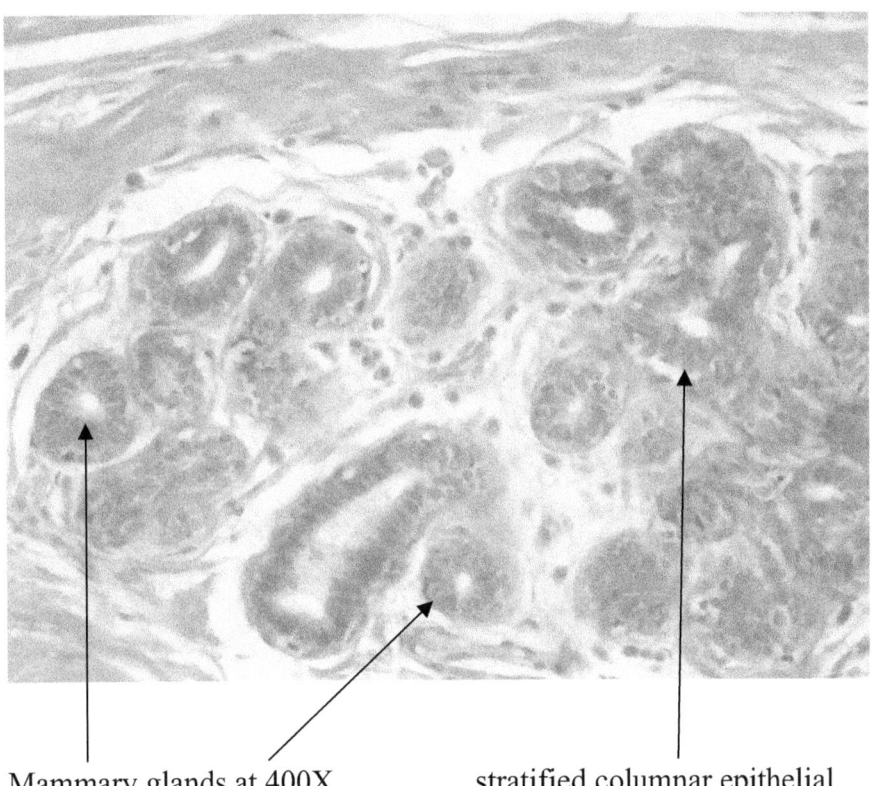

Mammary glands at 400X   stratified columnar epithelial

The mammary glands are the milk producing glands of the female.

MITOSIS

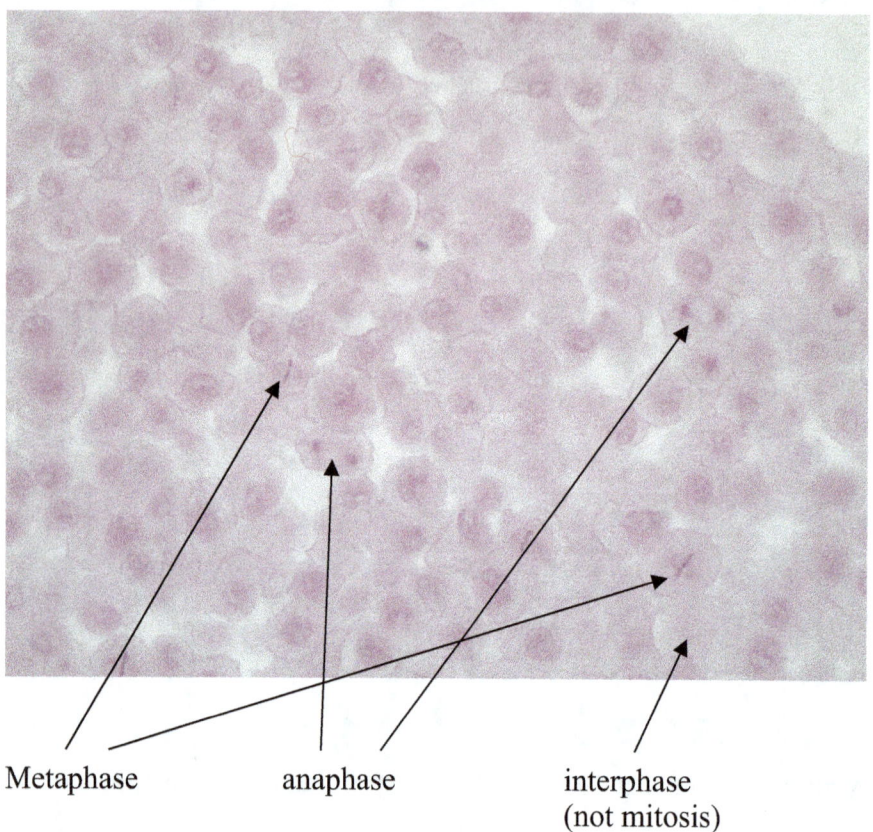

Metaphase   anaphase   interphase (not mitosis)

Mitosis at 400X

The cell life cycle is divided into interphase, mitosis, and cytokinesis.

Mitosis is divided into 4 phases: prophase, metaphase, anaphase, and telophase.

Metaphase is identified by the chromosomes lining up across the center (equator) of the cell.

Anaphase is identified by the splitting of the chromosomes.

MITOSIS

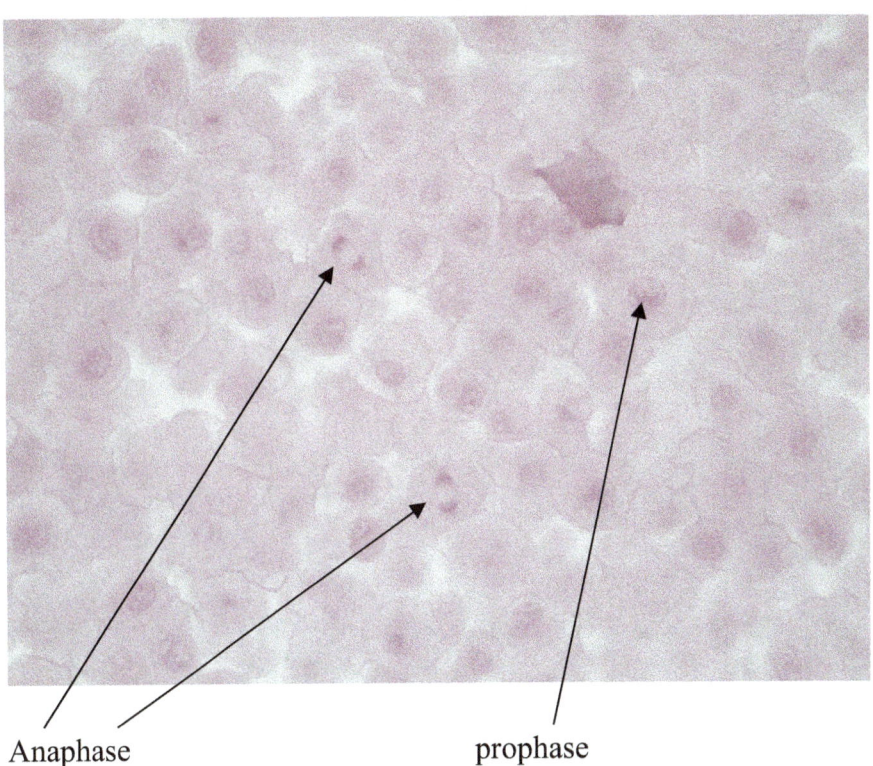

Anaphase   prophase

Mitosis at 400X

The cell life cycle is divided into interphase, mitosis, and cytokinesis.

Mitosis is divided into 4 phases: prophase, metaphase, anaphase, and telophase.

Anaphase is identified by the splitting of the chromosomes.

Prophase is identified by the appearance of the chromosomes.

MITOSIS

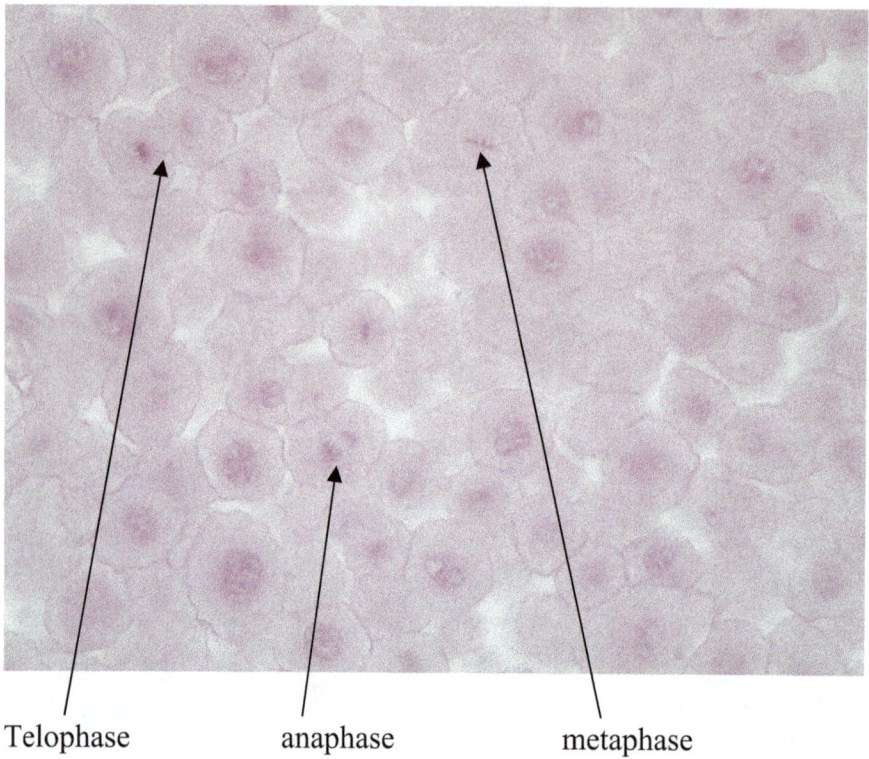

Telophase   anaphase   metaphase

Mitosis at 400X

The cell life cycle is divided into interphase, mitosis, and cytokinesis.

Mitosis is divided into 4 phases: prophase, metaphase, anaphase, and telophase.

Anaphase is identified by the splitting of the chromosomes.

Metaphase is identified by the chromosomes lining up across the center (equator) of the cell.

Telephase is identified by the splitting of the cells.

MITOSIS

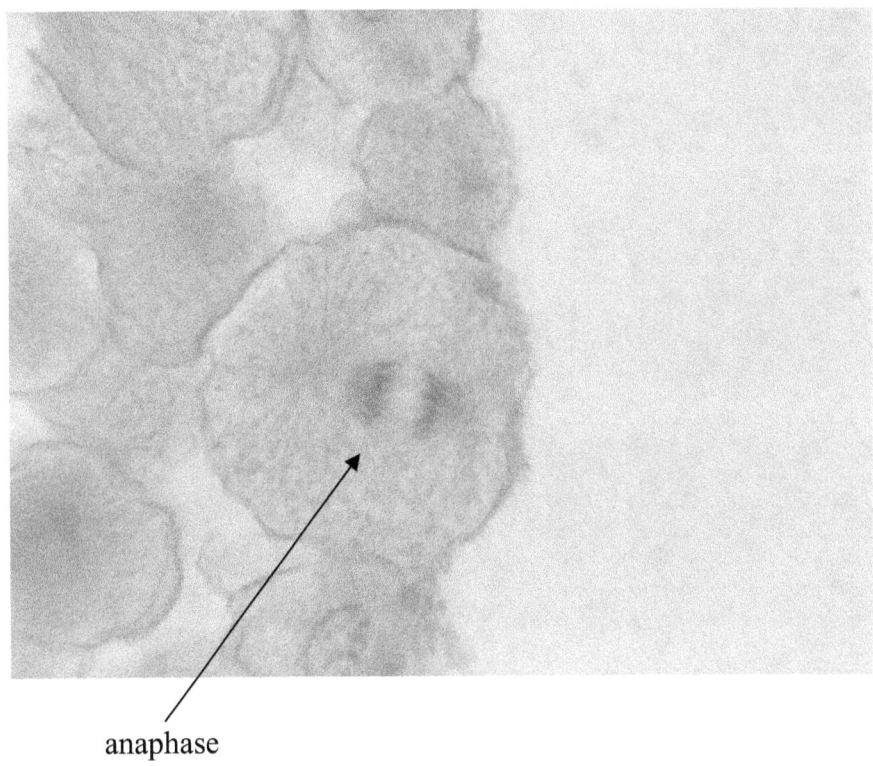

anaphase

Mitosis at 1000X

Notice the dividing of the nucleus.

Anaphase is identified by the splitting of the chromosomes.

MITOSIS

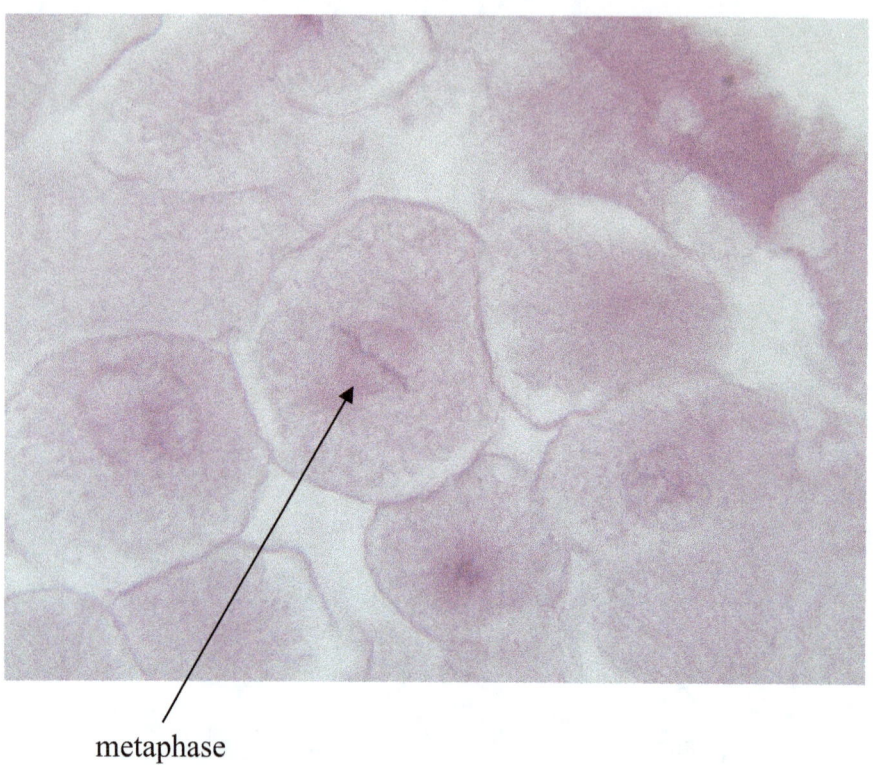

metaphase

Mitosis at 1000X

When the chromosomes are lined up at the equator (center) of the cell, metaphase is clearly visible.

MITOSIS

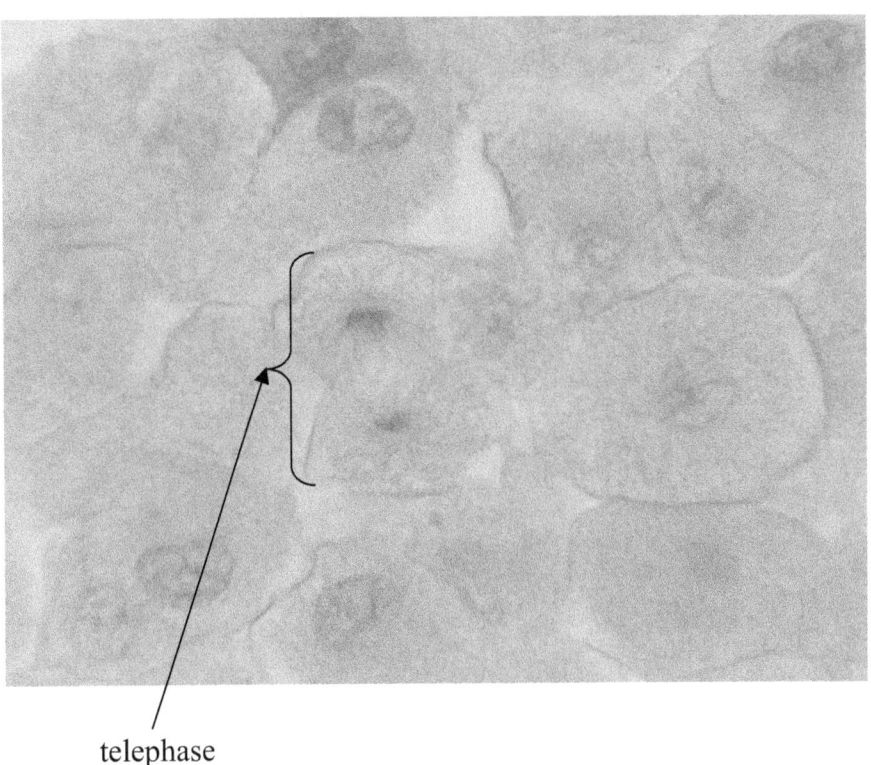

telephase

Mitosis at 1000X

Telophase is seen when the cells are dividing. This division of the cytoplasm is called cytokinesis.

Mitosis is division of the nucleus, but cytokinesis is division of the cytoplasm (everything else).

Telephase is identified by the splitting of the cells.

MOTOR END PLATES

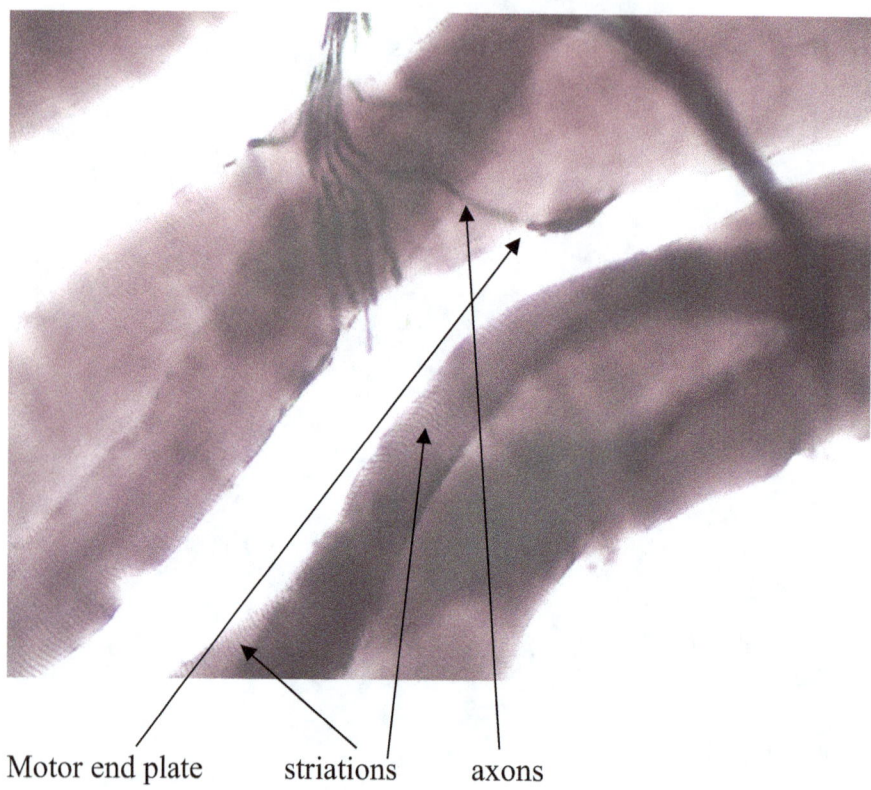

Motor end plate   striations   axons

Motor end plates at 400X

The motor end plates are the site of the neuromuscular junction. At the neuromuscular junction this is where a neuron communicates with a muscle or some other cell. A motor neuron will release acetylcholine where it meets a skeletal muscle. This acetylcholine will open ligand gated sodium channels, causing a depolarization. The depolarization will cause muscle contraction.

MOTOR END PLATES

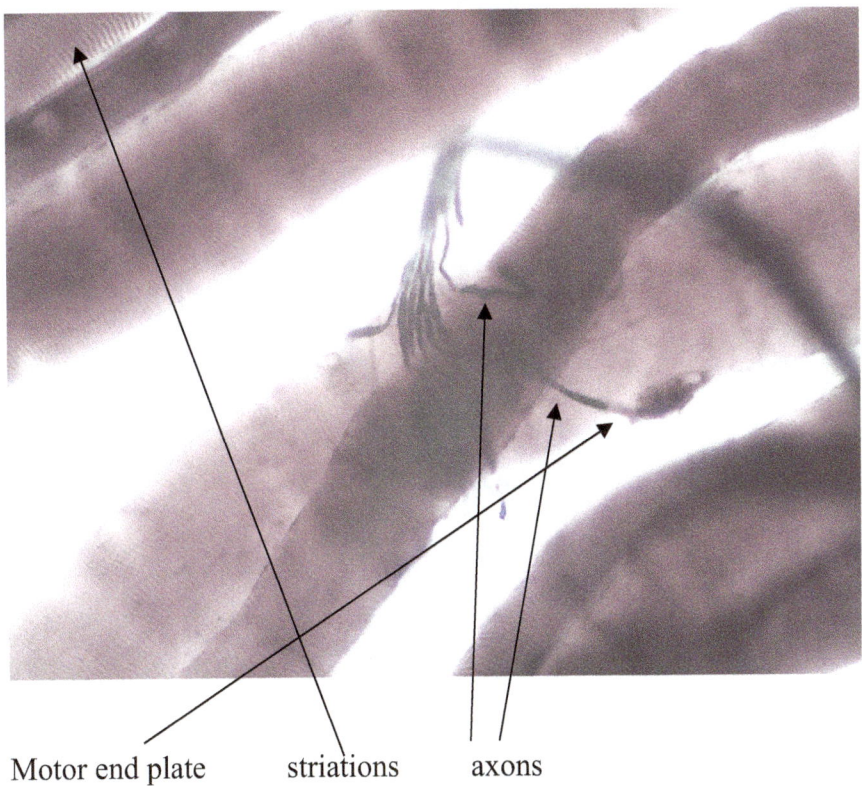

Motor end plate   striations   axons

Motor end plates at 400X

The motor end plates are the site of the neuromuscular junction. At the neuromuscular junction this is where a neuron communicates with a muscle or some other cell. A motor neuron will release acetylcholine where it meets a skeletal muscle. This acetylcholine will open ligand gated sodium channels, causing a depolarization. The depolarization will cause muscle contraction.

NERVE

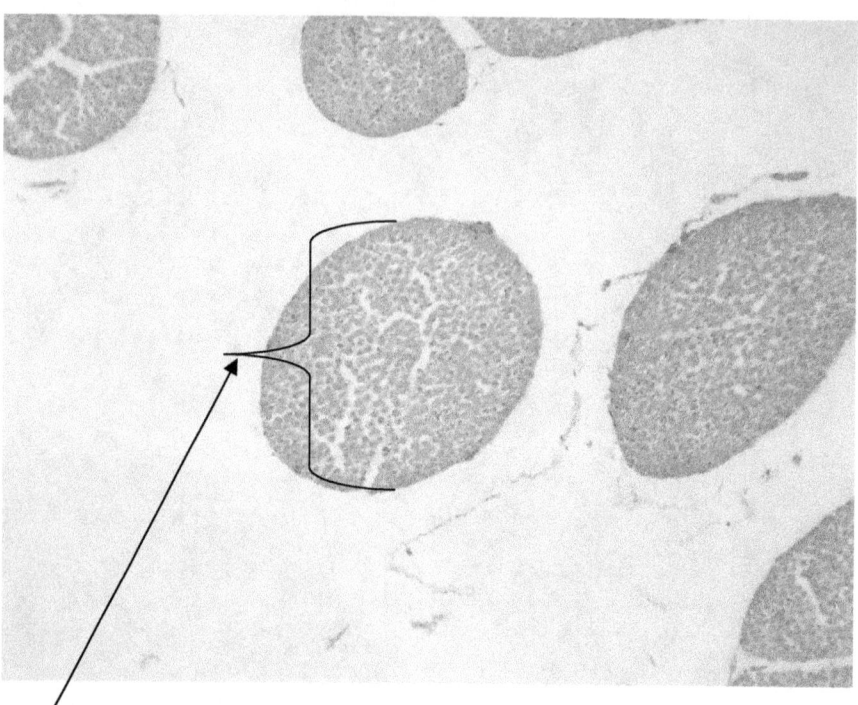

Nerve (bundle of axons)

Nerve at 40X

A nerve is a bundle of axons. Between the axons is myelin and this lipid material will act as insulation. This insulation is just like the rubber around a copper wire in any electric appliance. The insulation keeps electric signals (action potentials) in the axons and prevents them from going somewhere they shouldn't.

NERVE

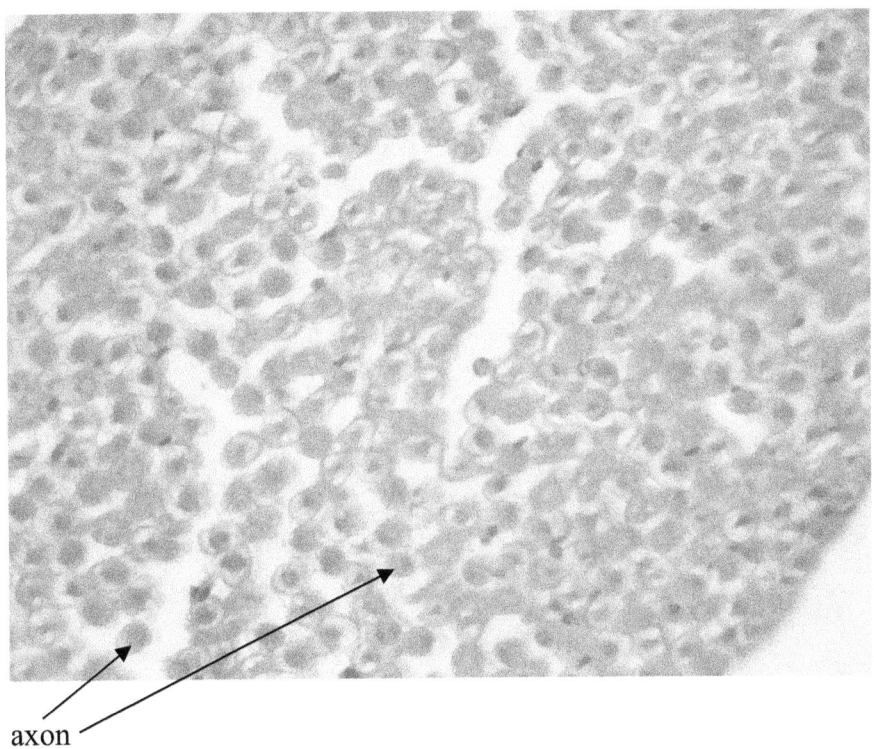

axon

Nerve at 100X

Cross sections of individual axons can be seen inside the nerve.

OVARY – MATURE FOLLICLE

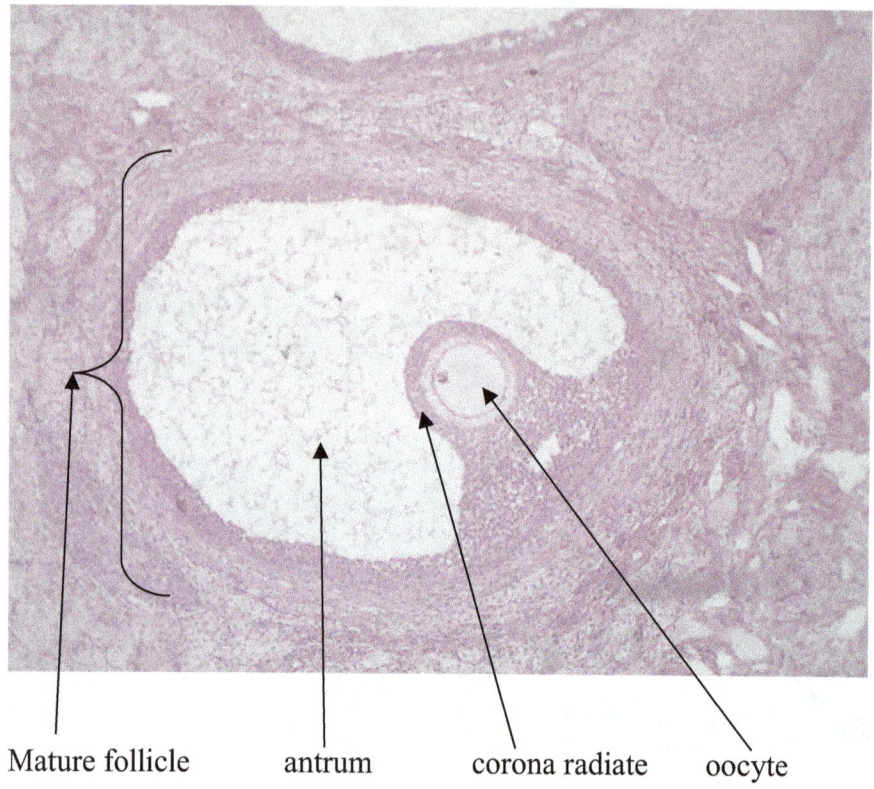

Mature follicle   antrum   corona radiate   oocyte

Ovary at 40X

The ovaries are the gonads of the female. The gonads are the organs responsible for producing the gametes (reproductive cells of the body).

Of the mature follicle above, only the oocyte plus a few layers of surrounding epithelial cells are released at the time of ovulation. Ovulation in the release of the oocyte from the ovaries.

The mature follicle is a collection of many cells and is the production site for estrogen and progesterone. The oocyte is a large cell seen within the mature follicle. A mature follicle is also called a Grafian follicle.

OVARY – MATURE FOLLICLE

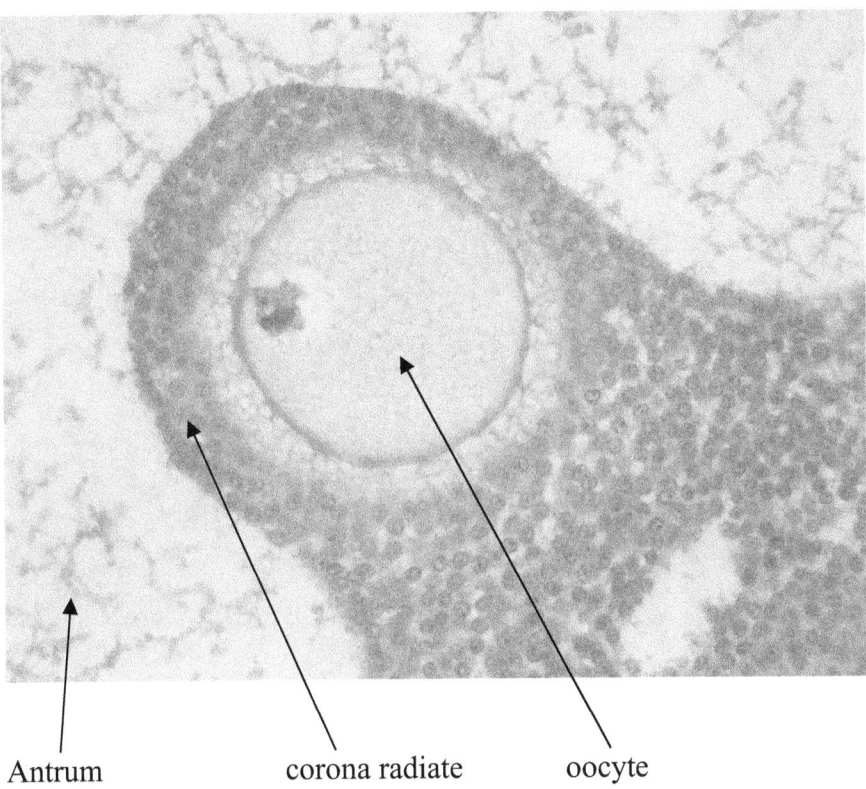

Antrum   corona radiate   oocyte

Ovary at 100X

Of the mature follicle above, only the oocyte plus a few layers of surrounding epithelial cells are released at the time of ovulation. Ovulation in the release of the oocyte from the ovaries.

The mature follicle is a collection of many cells and is the production site for estrogen and progesterone. The oocyte is a large cell seen within the mature follicle. A mature follicle is also called a Grafian follicle.

PANCREAS

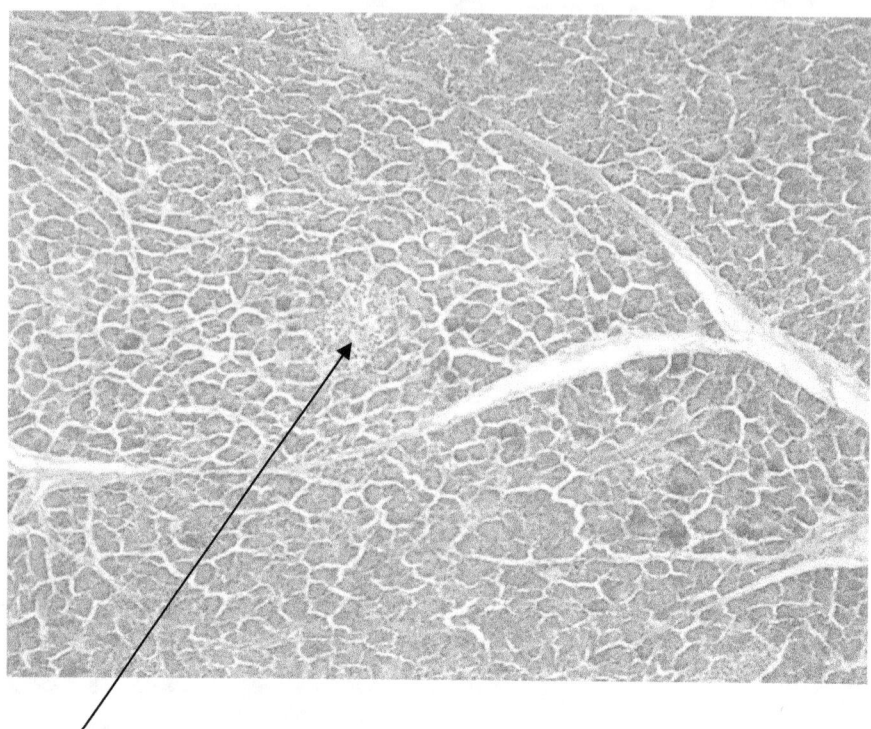

Pancreatic islets

Pancreas at 100X

The pancreatic islets are the endocrine portion of the pancreas. These groups of cells produce hormones like insulin and glucagon. These two hormones are responsible for maintaining our blood sugar levels.

PANCREAS

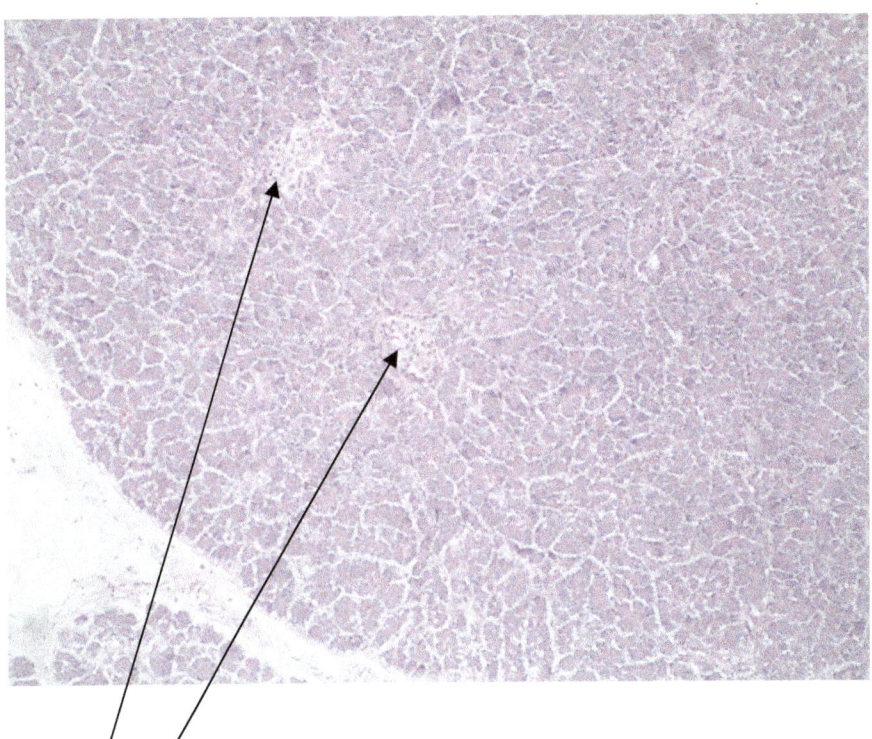

Pancreatic islets

Pancreas at 100X

The pancreas is a major part of the digestive system. The pancreas produces digestive enzymes for all the organic molecules human consume. These enzymes are released into the duodenum, which is the first part of the small intestine.

PANCREAS

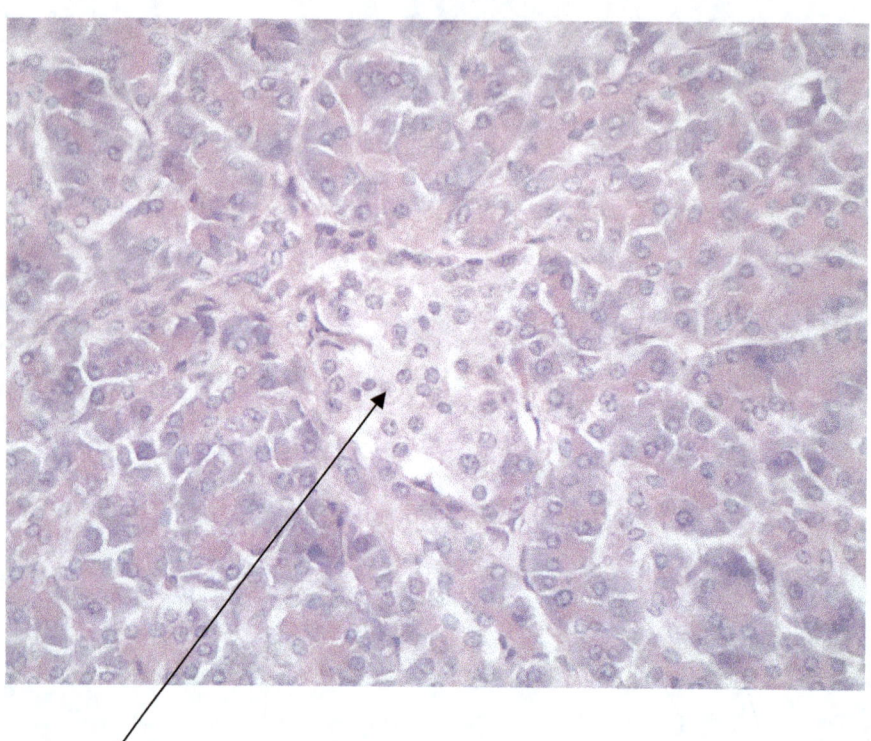

Pancreatic islet

Pancreas at 400X

PANCREAS

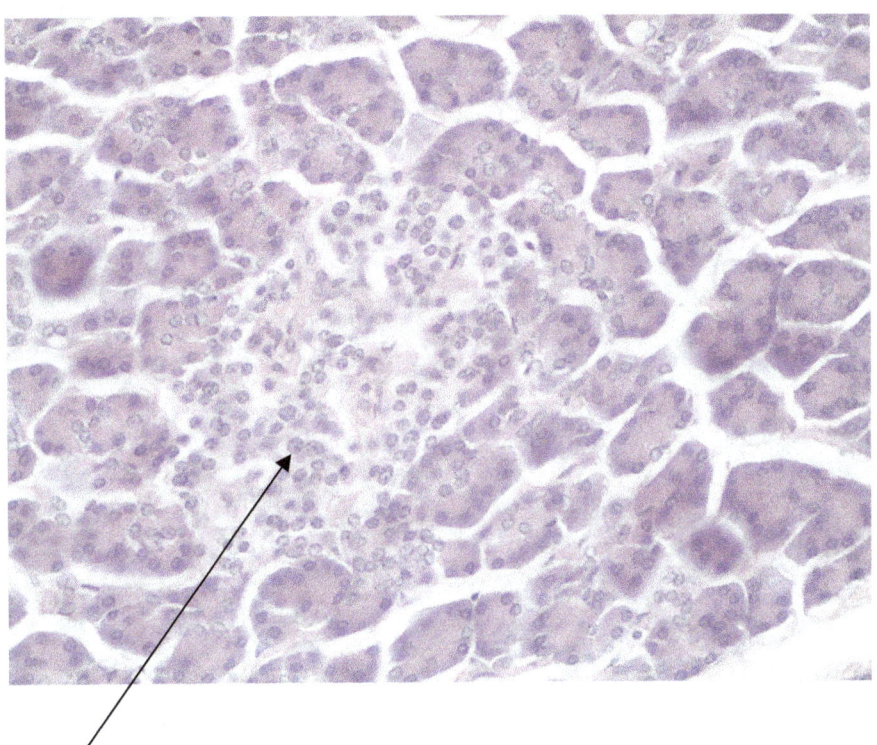

Pancreatic islet

Pancreas at 400X

PARATHYROID GLAND

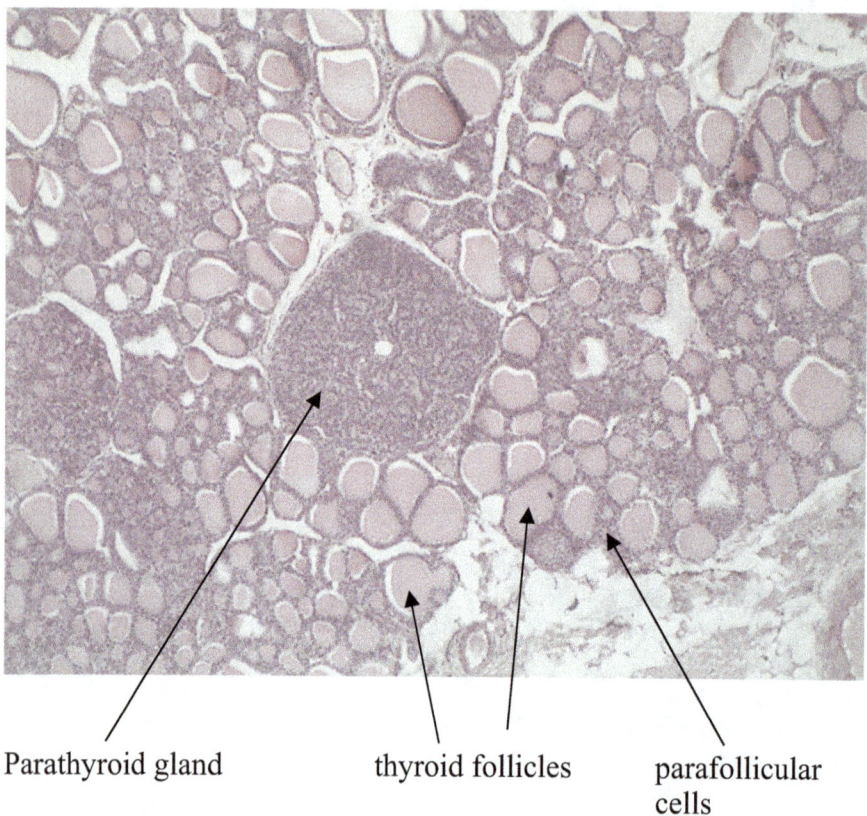

Parathyroid gland   thyroid follicles   parafollicular cells

Parathyroid gland at 100X

The parathyroid glands are found on the posterior surface of the thyroid gland and are responsible for producing and releasing parathyroid hormone (PTH). PTH works to raise blood calcium levels.

The thyroid follicles are part of the thyroid gland. These follicles are the storage sites for the hormones T3 andT4, which work to regulate metabolism.

PARATHYROID GLAND

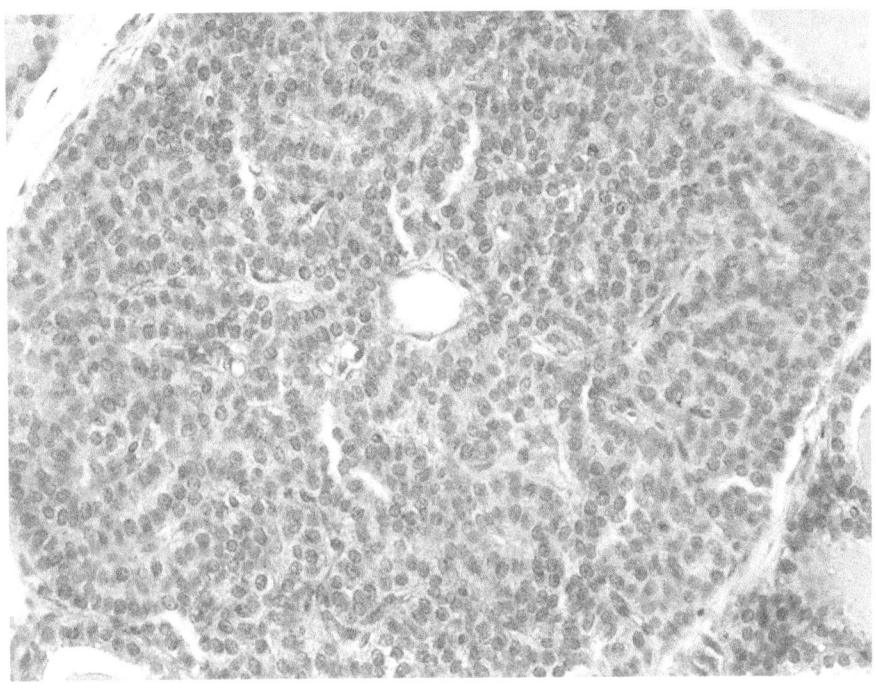

Parathyroid gland at 100X

The parathyroid glands are found on the posterior surface of the thyroid gland and are responsible for producing and releasing parathyroid hormone (PTH). PTH works to raise blood calcium levels.

PITUITARY GLAND (anterior)

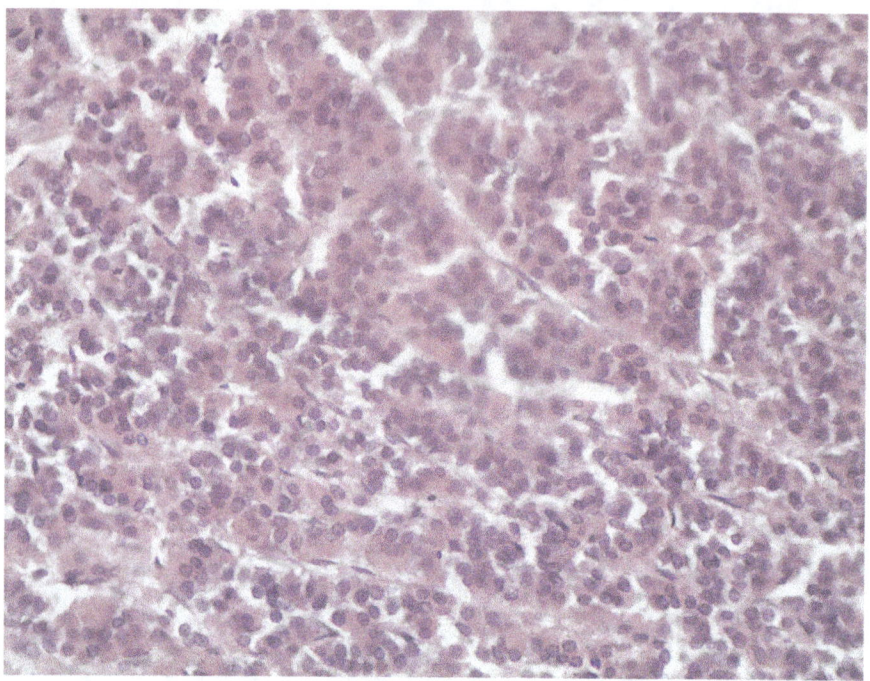

Pituitary gland at 400X

See hypophysis for more pictures.

The pituitary gland has 2 halves the anterior (adenohypophysis) and the posterior (neurohypophysis). The anterior half is made of epithelial cells and these cells produce 9 major hormones.

PROSTATE GLAND

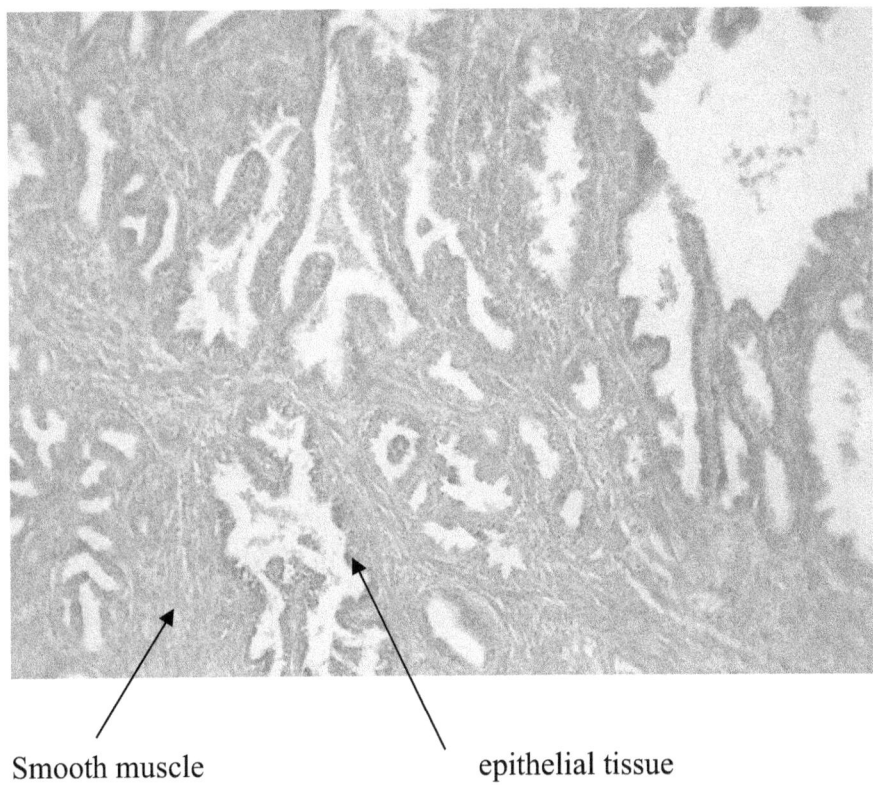

Smooth muscle   epithelial tissue

Prostate gland at 40X

The prostate gland is a singular gland found only in the male. This gland produces about 30% of the components of semen.

PROSTATE GLAND

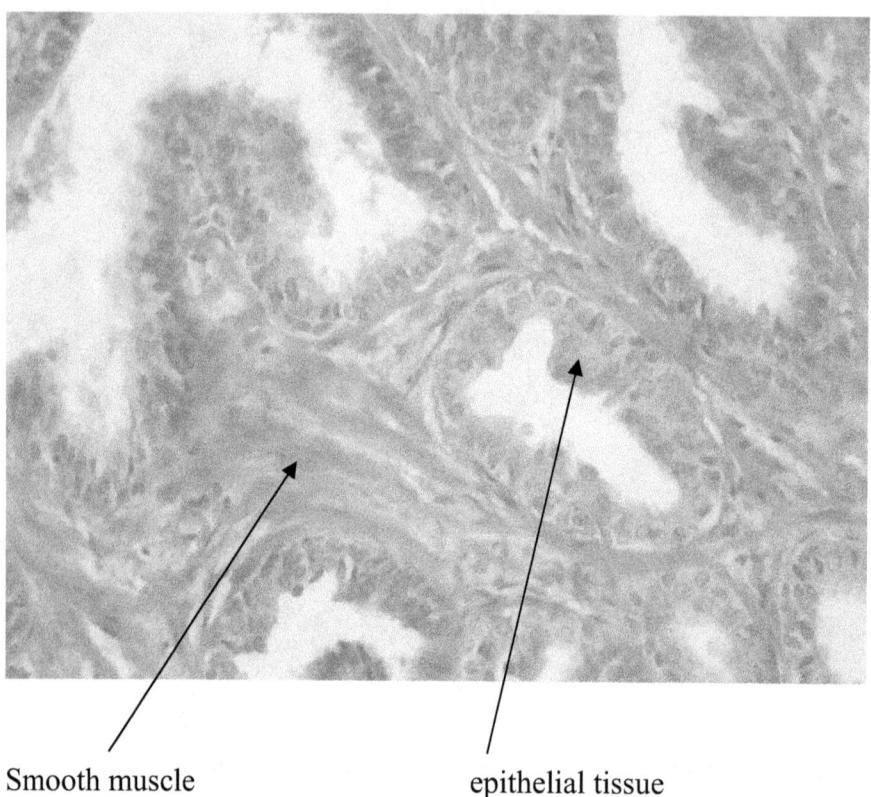

Smooth muscle   epithelial tissue

Prostate gland at 100X

RECTUM

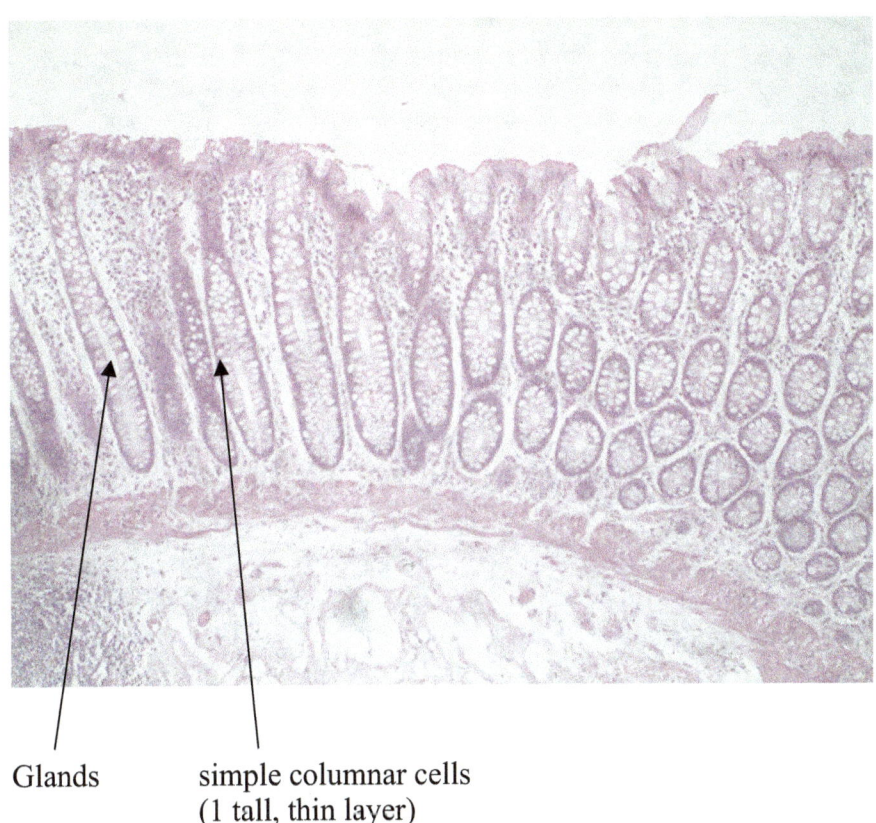

Glands   simple columnar cells
(1 tall, thin layer)

Rectum at 100X

Simple columnar cells are one tall, thin layer of epithelial cells.

RECTUM

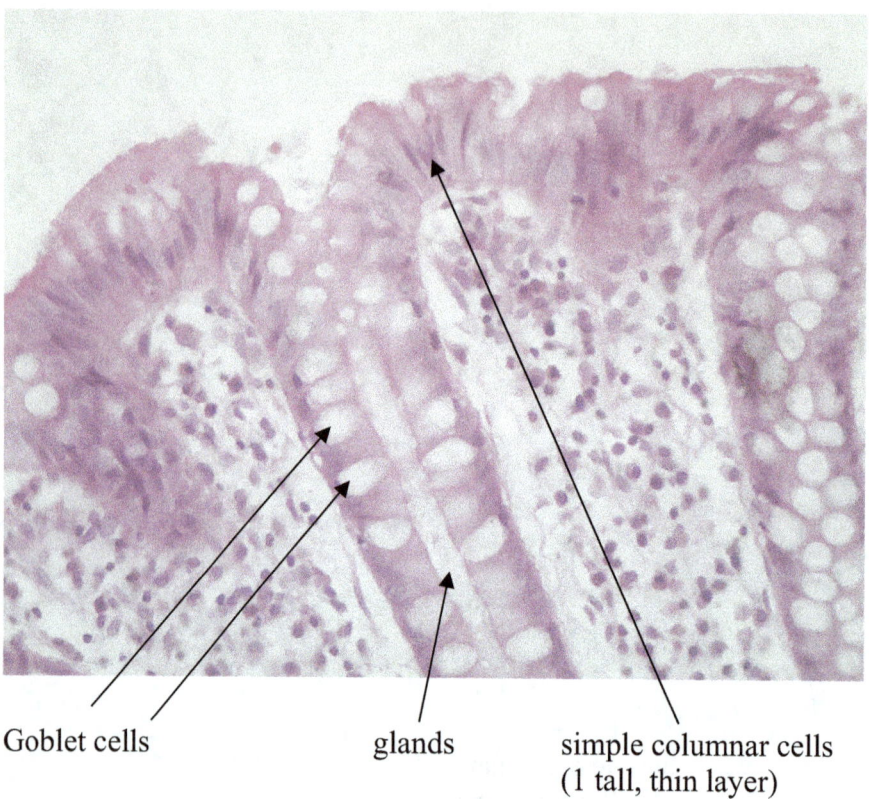

Goblet cells   glands   simple columnar cells
                                  (1 tall, thin layer)

Rectum at 400X

Goblet cells are the mucous producing cells of the body.

SCALP

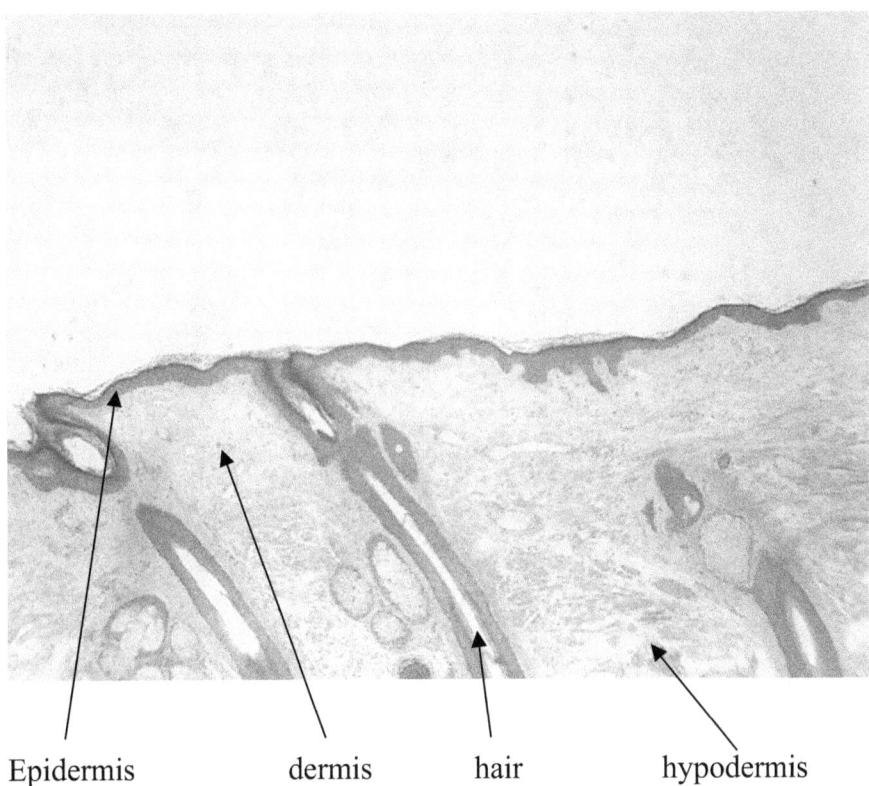

Epidermis   dermis   hair   hypodermis

Scalp at 40X

The scalp like the skin consists of two layers, the epidermis and dermis. The epidermis is the outer layer and consists of five strata (layers). The dermis is the deeper layer and consists of two layers. The epidermis is the outer stratified squamous layer we see on the surface. The dermis is the deeper layer where most of the strength is found in the skin.
Hairs can be seen in this picture. Hairs are places where the epidermis penetrates deep into the dermal layer.

SCALP

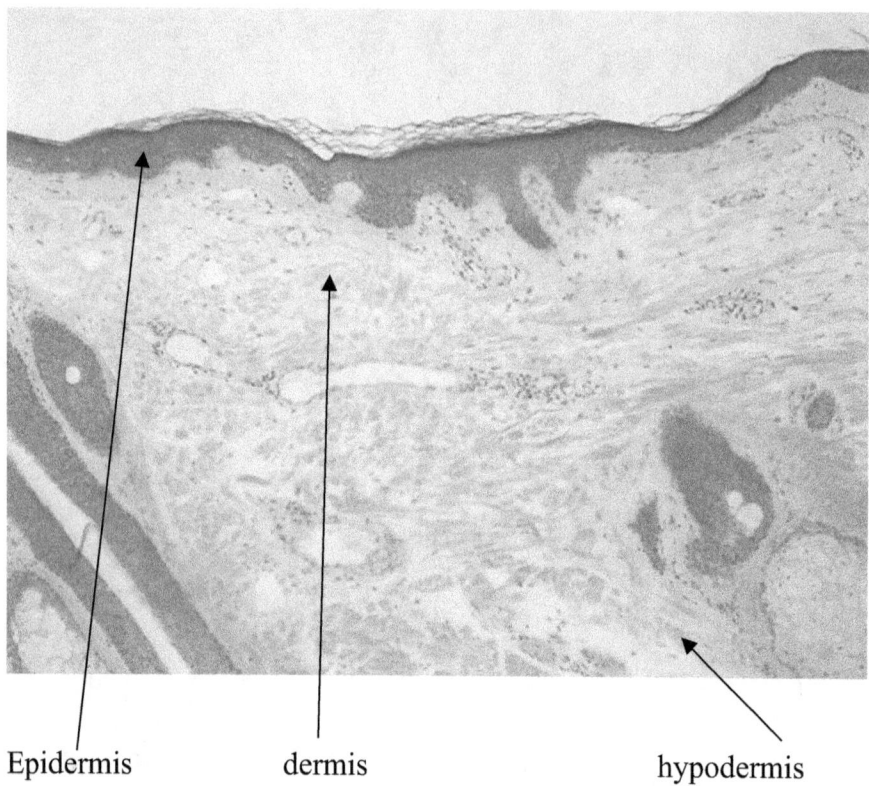

Epidermis   dermis   hypodermis

Scalp at 100X

Notice how much thicker the dermis is in comparison to the epidermis. The dermis is filled with collagen fibers, and this is where most of the strength of the skin is found.

The hypodermis is filled with adipose tissue.

SCALP

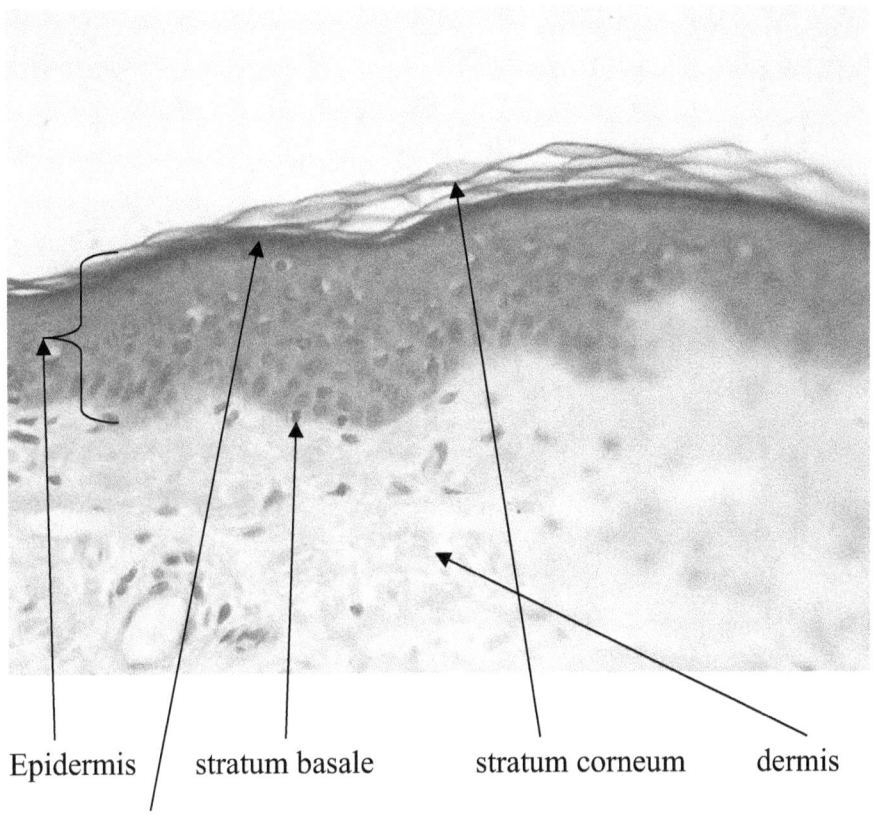

Epidermis / stratum basale   stratum corneum   dermis

Stratum granulosum

Scalp at 400X

Look at the superficial layer of the epidermis and notice how the cells are obviously squamous (flat) in shape.

SIMPLE COLUMNAR

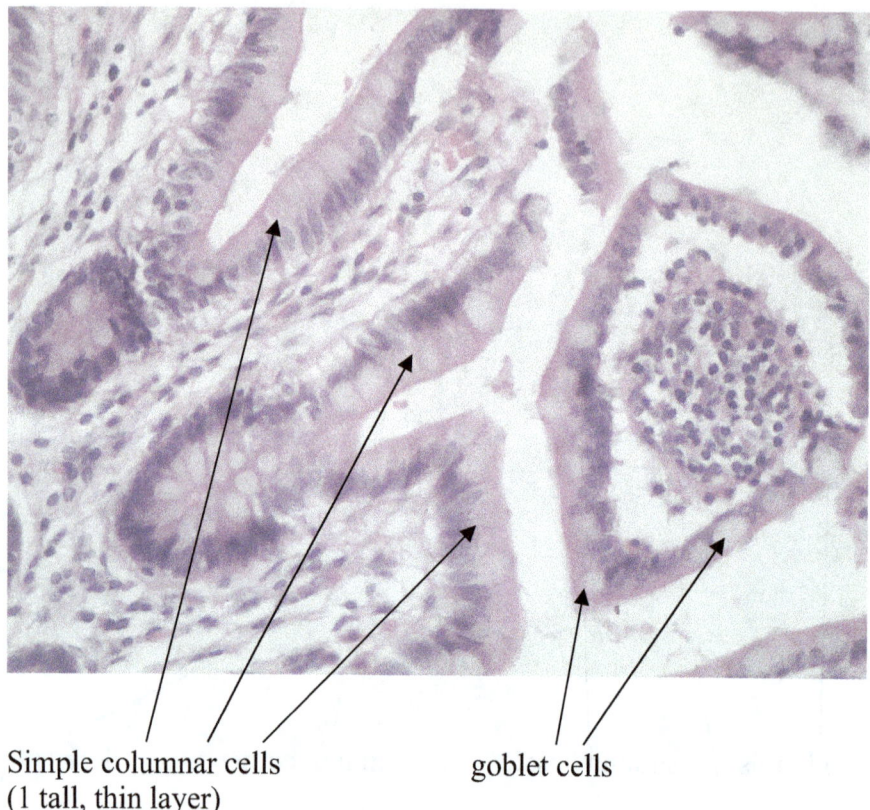

Simple columnar cells
(1 tall, thin layer)

goblet cells

Simple columnar at 400X

A simple columnar layer is one layer of tall, thin epithelial cells.

Goblet cells are mucous producing cells.

SIMPLE COLUMNAR

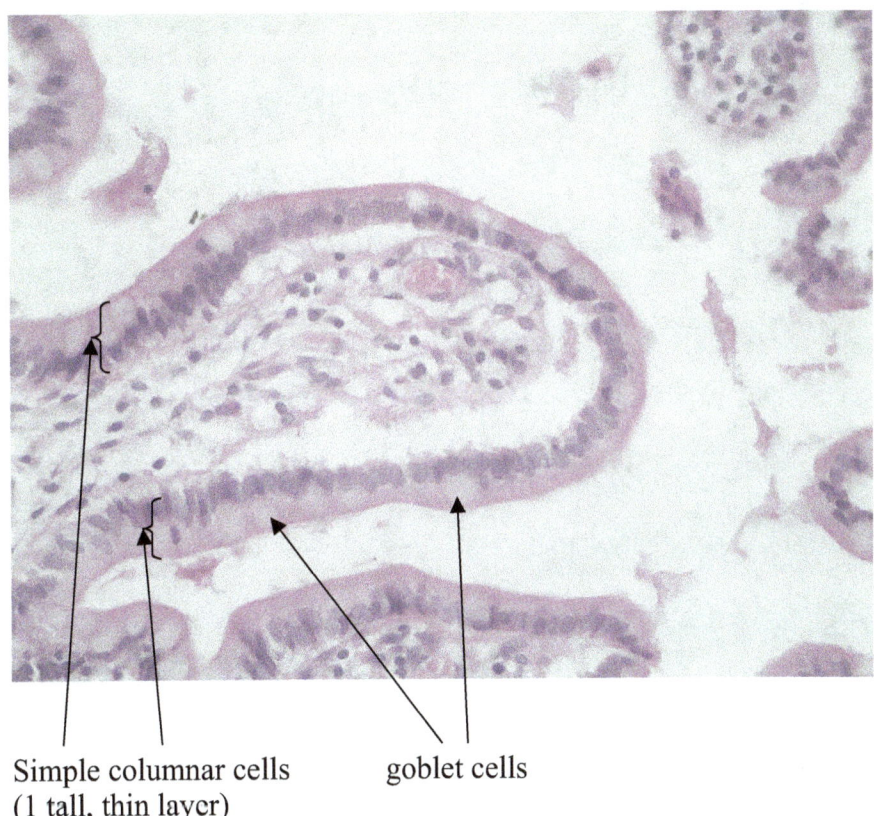

Simple columnar cells
(1 tall, thin layer)

goblet cells

Simple columnar at 400X

A simple columnar layer is one layer of tall, thin epithelial cells.

Goblet cells are mucous producing cells.

SKELETAL MUSCLE

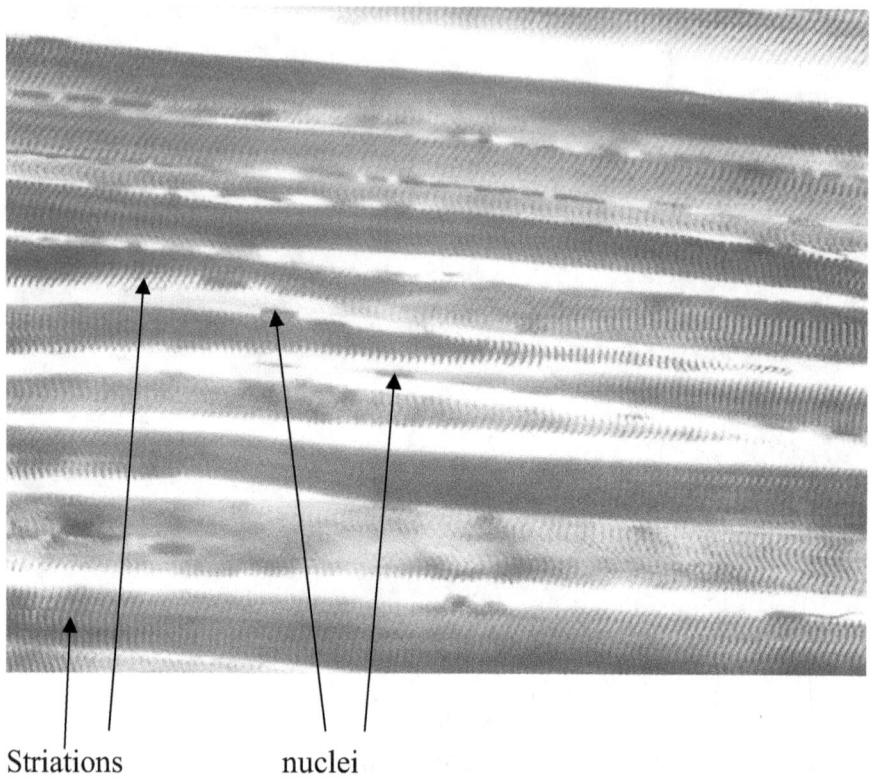

Striations   nuclei

Skeletal muscle at 400X

Skeletal muscle gets its name because it is always attached to one or more bones. Skeletal muscle is under voluntary control and has notable striations (stripes). The cells are long, cylinder shaped and multinucleated. They are responsible for body movement and about the only thing in the body we have conscious control over.

SKELETAL MUSCLE

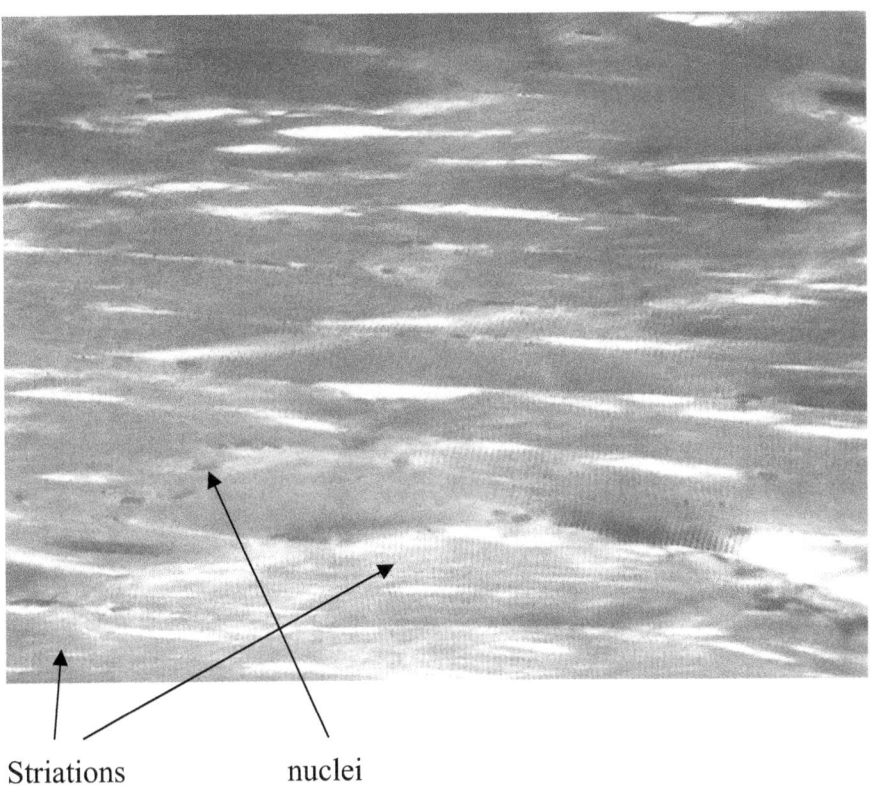

Striations   nuclei

Skeletal muscle at 400X

Notice the striations, this is a way to easily identify a longitudinal section of skeletal muscle.

SKELETAL MUSCLE and ARTERY

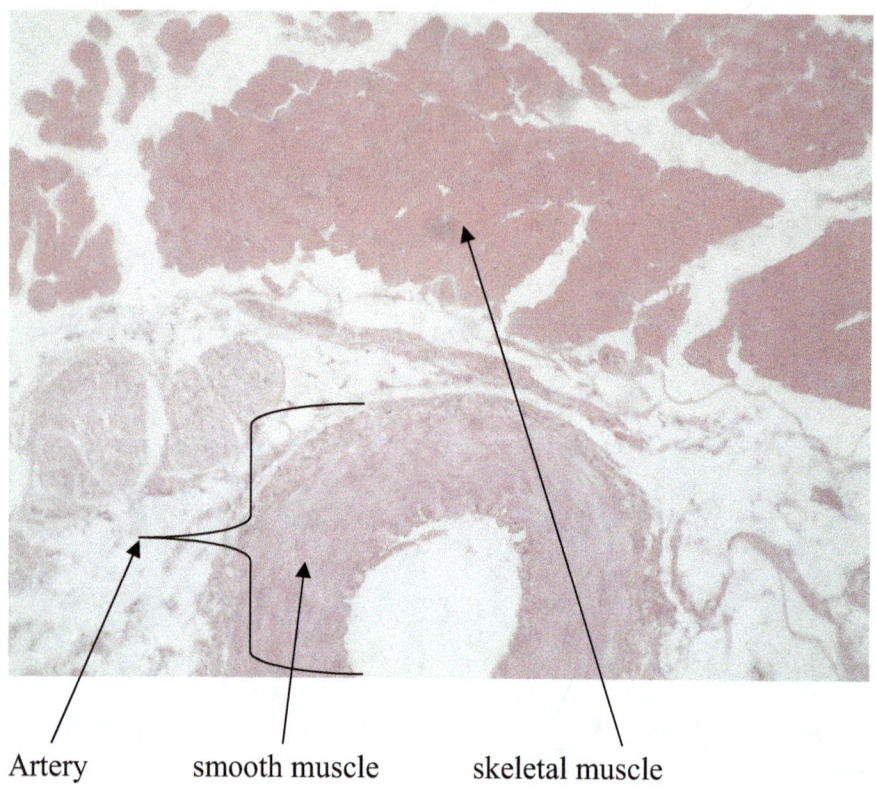

Artery   smooth muscle   skeletal muscle

Skeletal muscle and artery at 100X

In the cross section of skeletal muscle, you can't see the striations.

SKELETAL MUSCLE

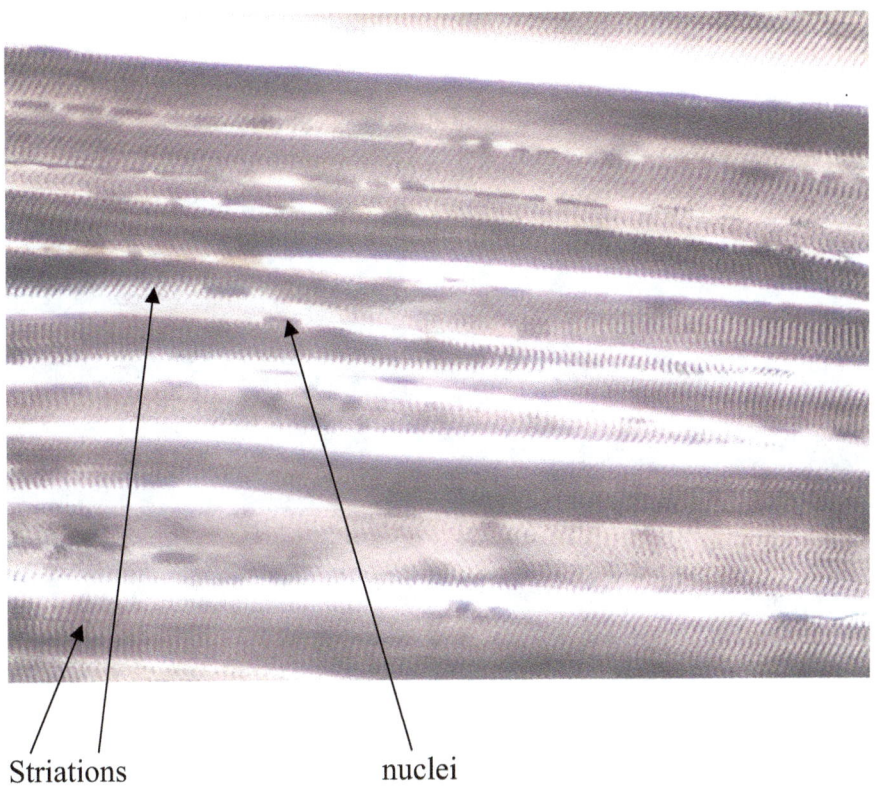

Striations   nuclei

Skeletal muscle at 400X

Notice the striations, this is a way to easily identify a longitudinal section of skeletal muscle. If you see these stripes, you think skeletal muscle.

SKIN

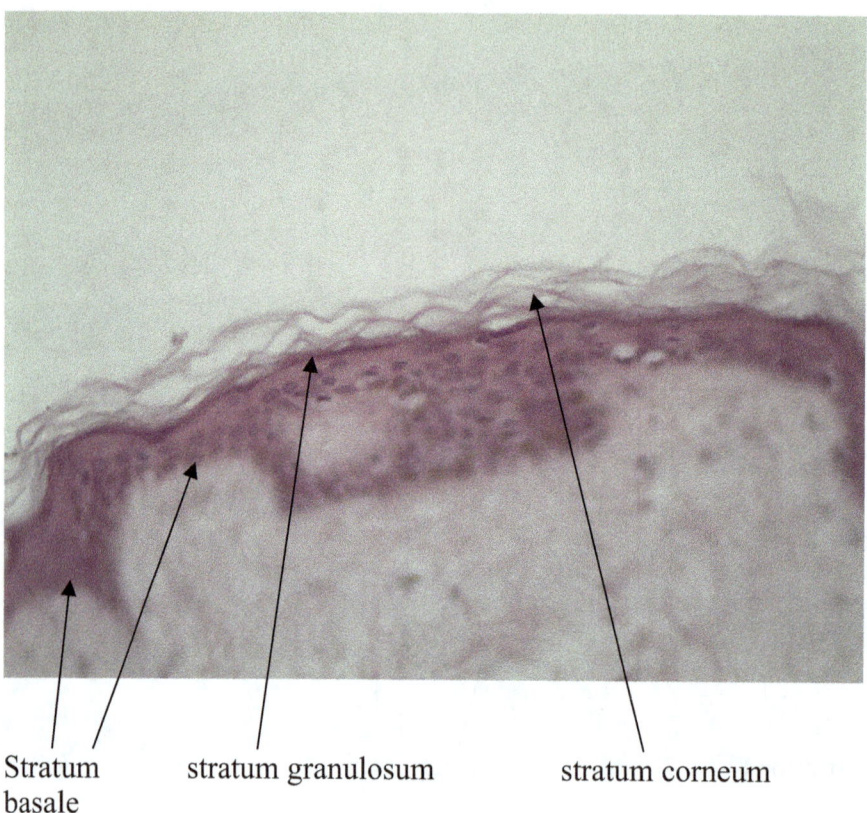

Stratum basale   stratum granulosum   stratum corneum

Skin at 400X

The skin consists of two layers, the epidermis and dermis. The epidermis is the outer layer and consists of five strata (layers). The dermis is the deeper layer and consists of two strata.
The epidermis is the outer stratified squamous layer we see on the surface. The dermis is the deeper layer where most of the strength is found in the skin.

SKIN

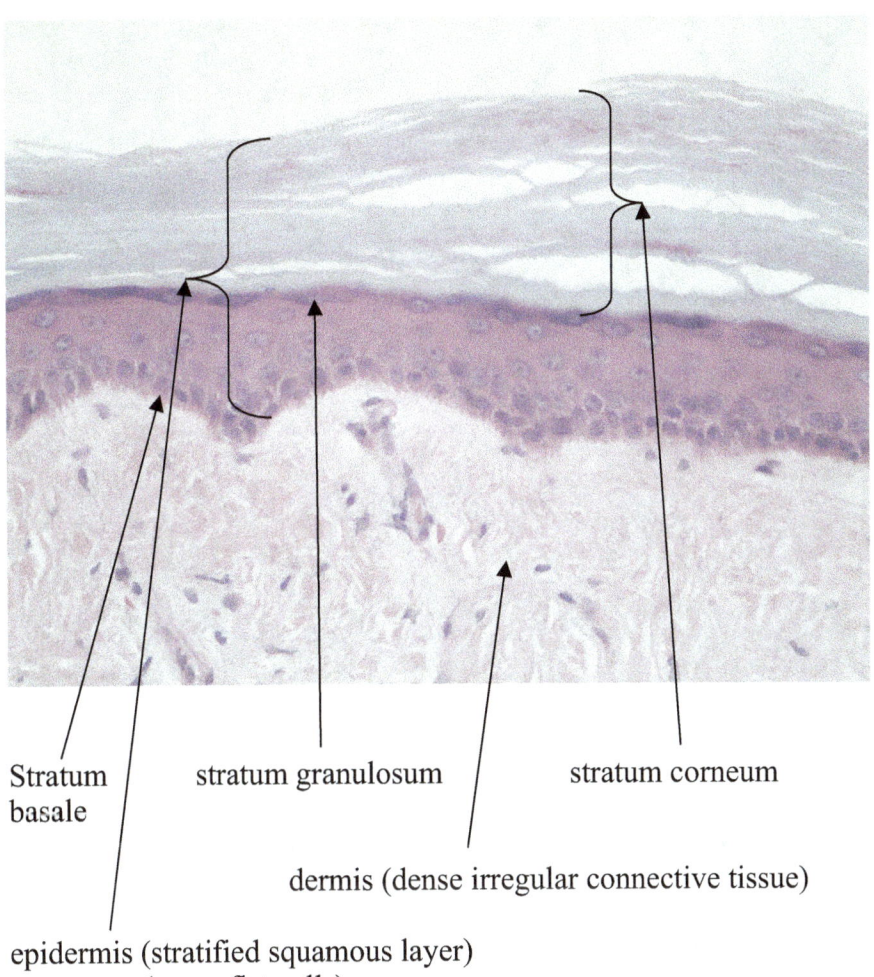

Stratum basale
stratum granulosum
stratum corneum
dermis (dense irregular connective tissue)
epidermis (stratified squamous layer) (many flat cells)

Skin at 400X

The epidermis is the outer layer of the skin, and the dermis is the deeper layer. The dermis is much thicker than the epidermis and is where most of the strength of the skin is found.

SMOOTH MUSCLE

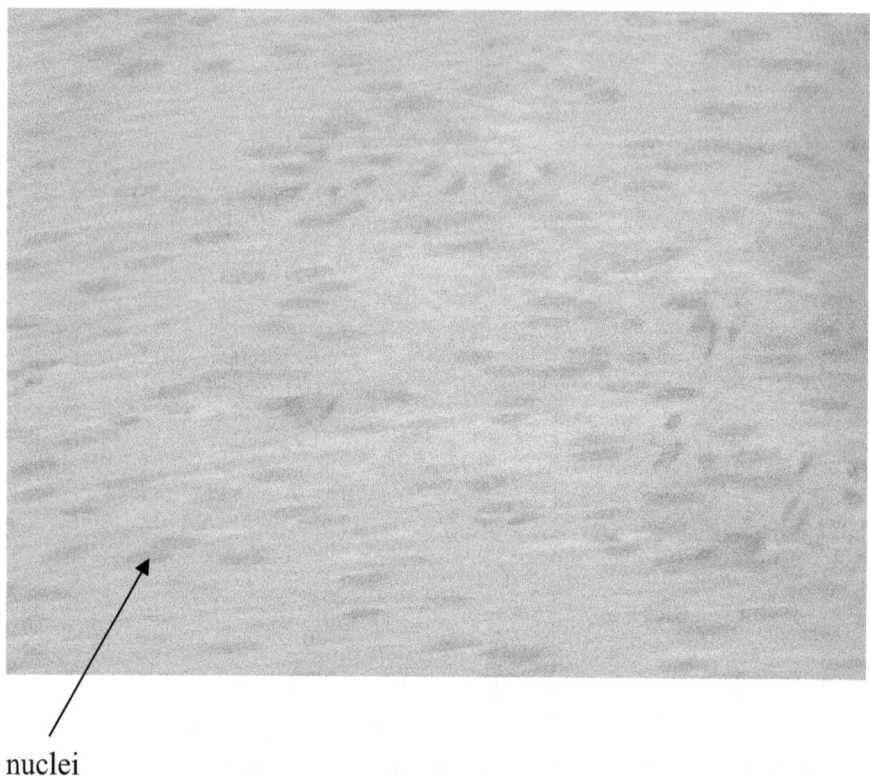

nuclei

Smooth muscle at 400X

Smooth muscle has a spindle shape, meaning it is thick in the center and thin at the edges (like a football). This muscle is involuntary and has a single nucleus. Smooth muscle is found in many places of the body, like around blood vessels, GI tract, urinary bladder, and pupil.

SMOOTH MUSCLE

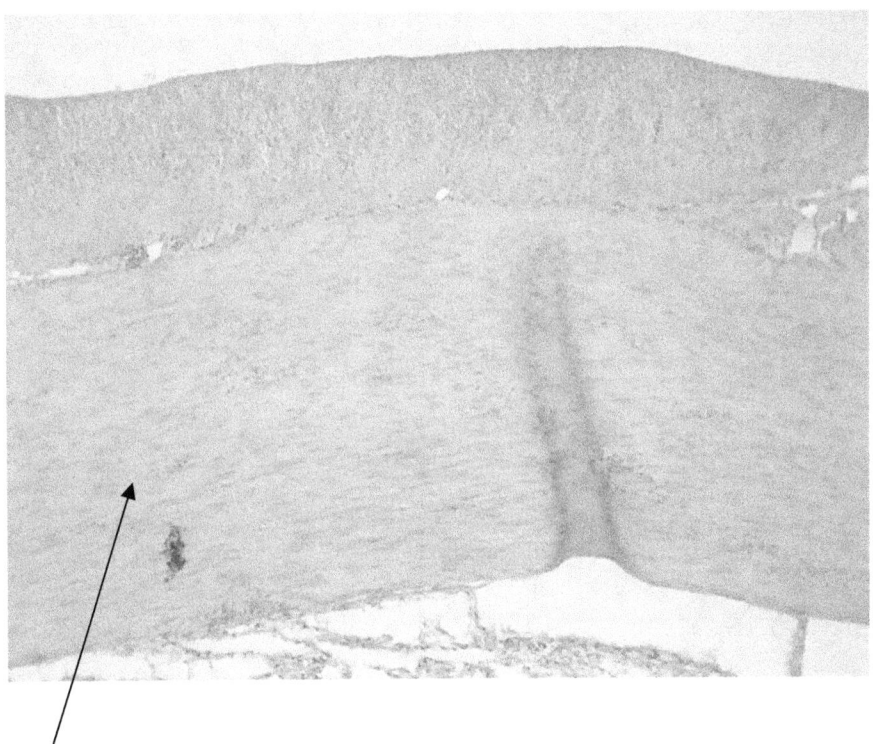

Smooth muscle

Smooth muscle from the ileum at 100X

Smooth muscle has a spindle shape, meaning it is thick in the center and thin at the edges (like a football). This muscle is involuntary and has a single nucleus. Smooth muscle is found in many places of the body like around blood vessels, GI tract, urinary bladder, and pupil.

SMOOTH MUSCLE

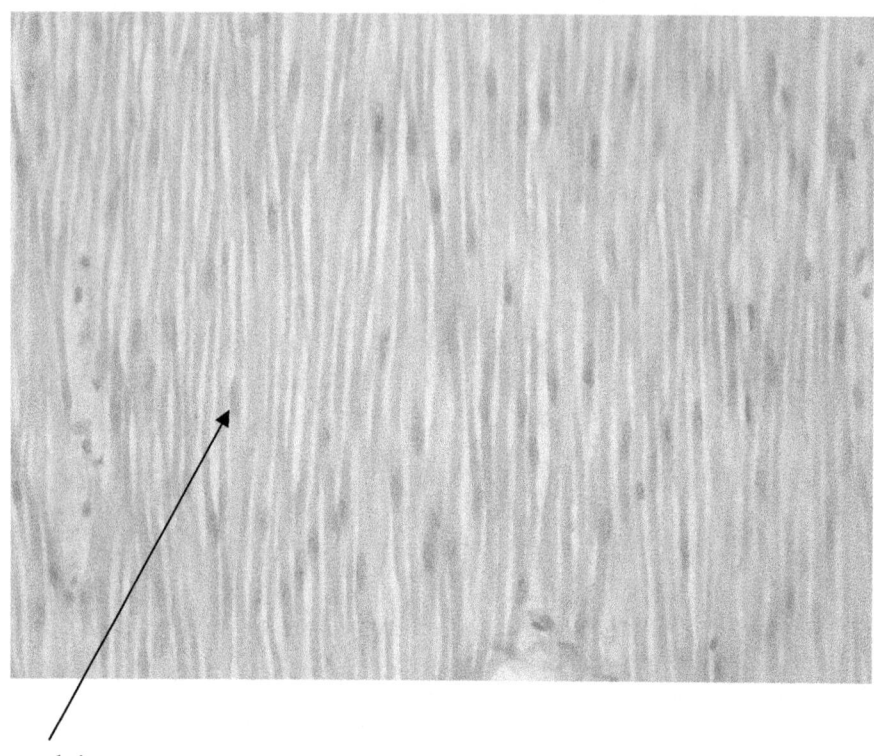

nuclei

Smooth muscle at 400X

Notice the cell layers are arranged from the top to the bottom of the slide picture.

Smooth muscle has a spindle shape, meaning it is thick in the center and thin at the edges (like a football). This muscle is involuntary and has a single nucleus. Smooth muscle is found in many places of the body like around blood vessels, GI tract, urinary bladder, and pupil.

SPINAL CORD

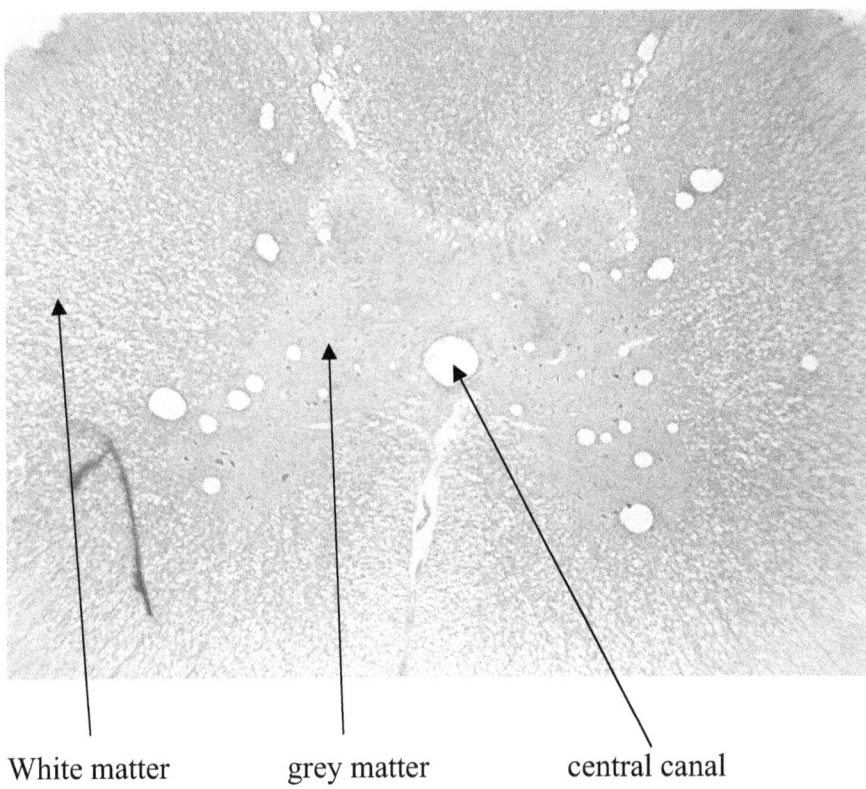

White matter   grey matter   central canal

Spinal cord at 40X

The spinal cord is part of the central nervous system and is found down the center of most of the vertebrae.

The spinal cord is made of an outer white matter region. This region is composed of mylineated axons.

The inner region is composed of grey matter. This region is composed of neuron cell bodies and dendrites.

In the center of the spinal cord is the central canal, where cerebrospinal fluid moves.

SPINAL CORD

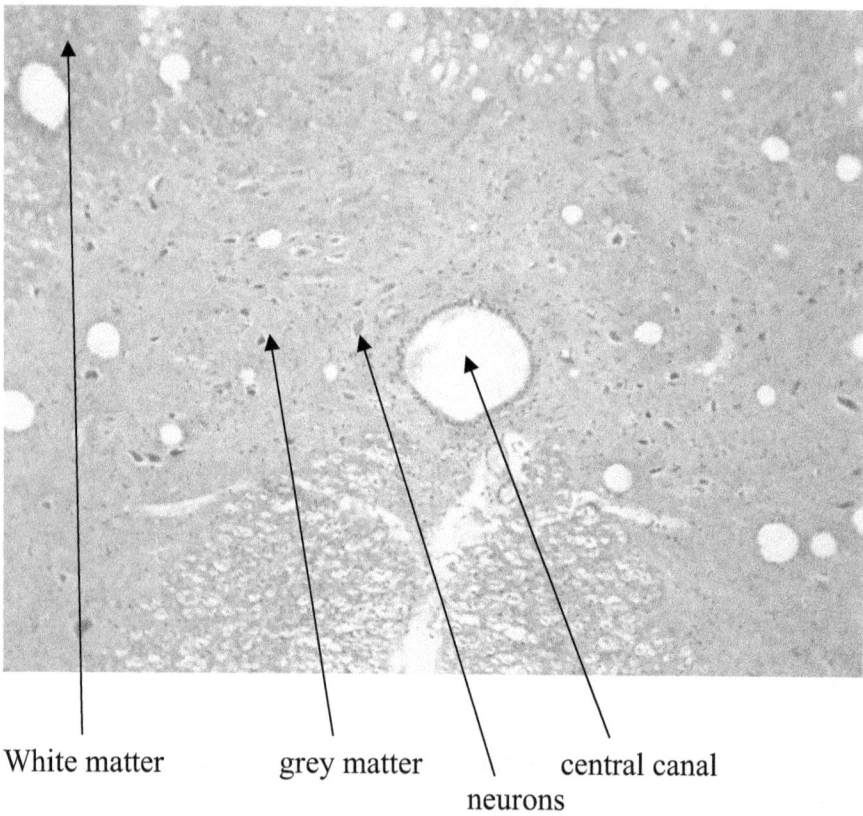

White matter   grey matter   central canal
                              neurons

Spinal cord at 100X

The spinal cord is part of the central nervous system and is found down the center of most of the vertebrae.

The spinal cord is made of an outer white matter region. This region is composed of mylineated axons.

The inner region is composed of grey matter. This region is composed of neuron cell bodies and dendrites.

In the center of the spinal cord is the central canal, where cerebrospinal fluid moves.

SPINAL CORD

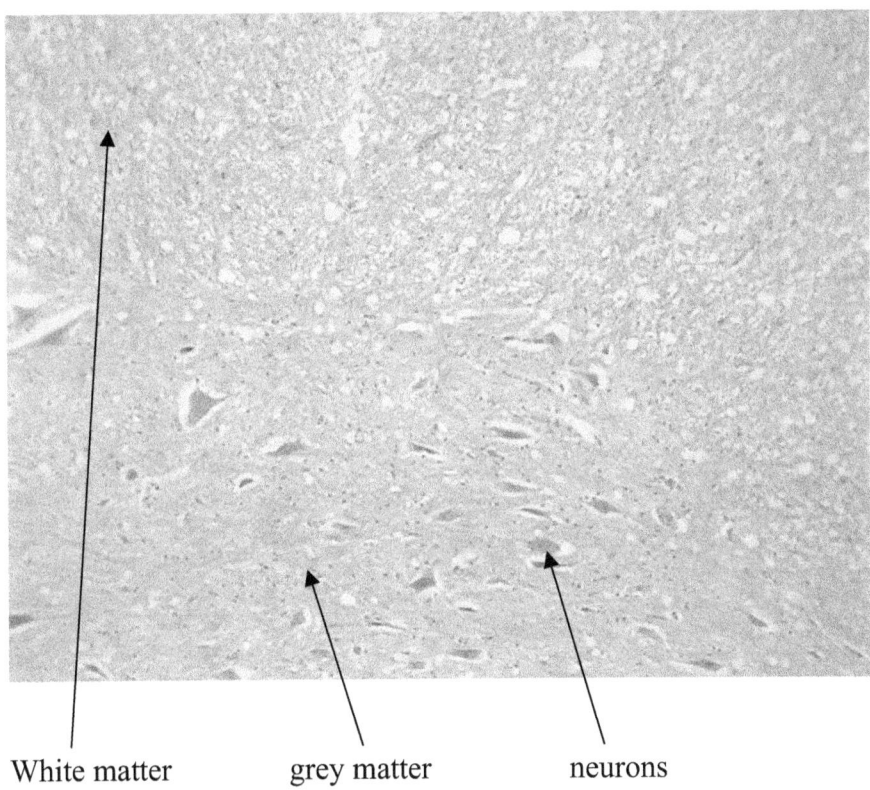

White matter   grey matter   neurons

Spinal cord at 100X

The spinal cord is part of the central nervous system and is found down the center of most of the vertebrae.

The spinal cord is made of an outer white matter region. This region is composed of mylineated axons.

The inner region is composed of grey matter. This region is composed of neuron cell bodies and dendrites.

In the center of the spinal cord is the central canal, where cerebrospinal fluid moves.

SPINAL CORD

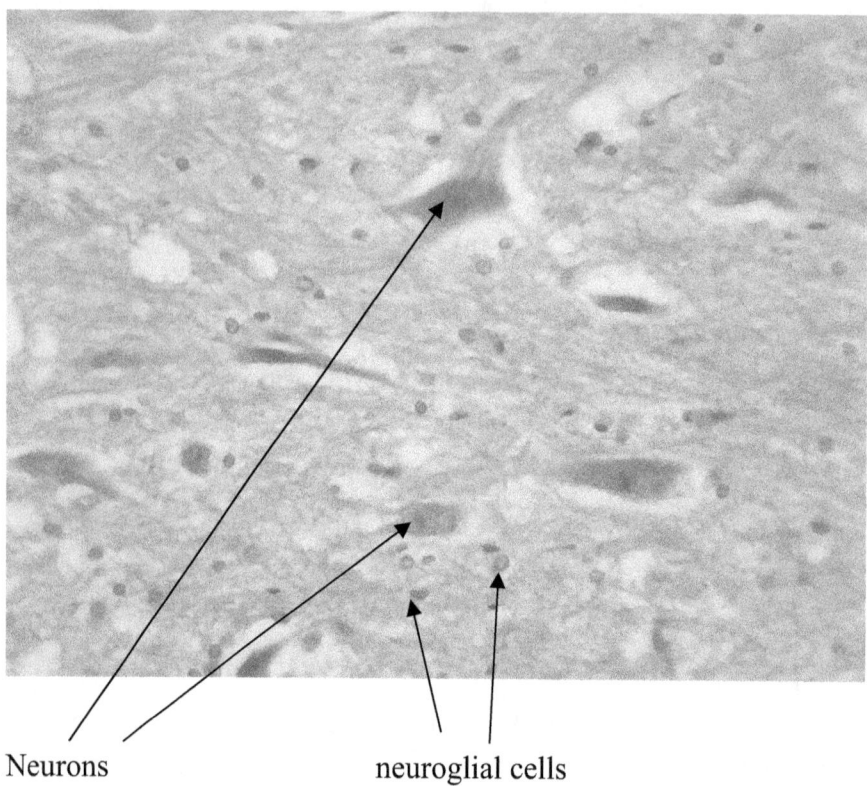

Neurons   neuroglial cells

Spinal cord at 400X

The spinal cord is part of the central nervous system and is found down the center of most of the vertebrae.

The spinal cord is made of an outer white matter region. This region is composed of mylineated axons.

The inner region is composed of grey matter. This region is composed of neuron cell bodies and dendrites.

In the center of the spinal cord is the central canal, where cerebrospinal fluid moves.

SPINAL CORD

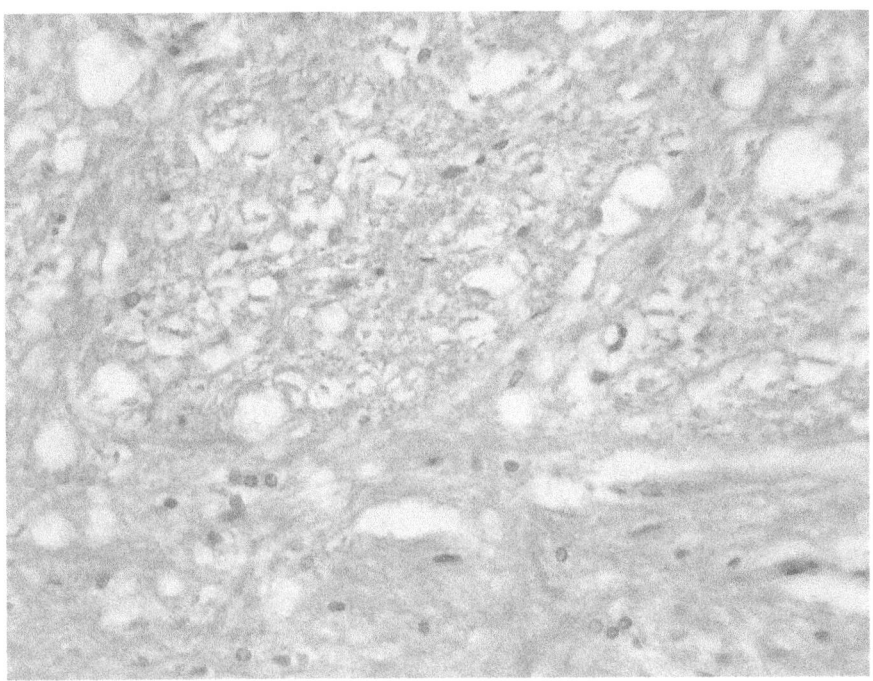

Spinal cord at 400X

The spinal cord is part of the central nervous system and is found down the center of most of the vertebrae.

The spinal cord is made of an outer white matter region. This region is composed of mylineated axons.

The inner region is composed of grey matter. This region is composed of neuron cell bodies and dendrites.

In the center of the spinal cord is the central canal, where cerebrospinal fluid moves.

SPINAL CORD

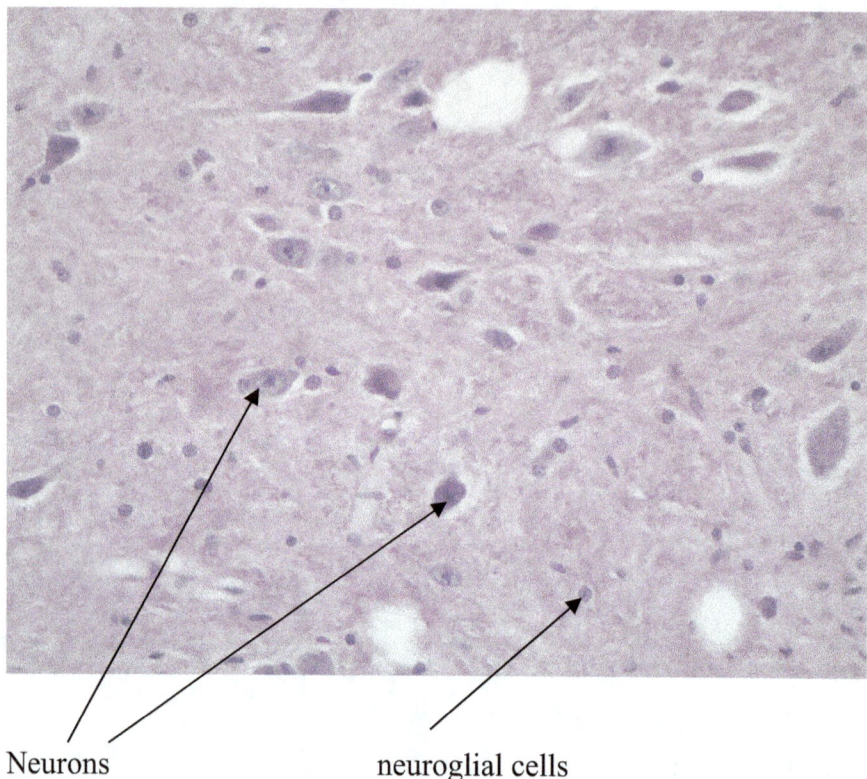

Neurons   neuroglial cells

Spinal cord (grey matter) at 400X

The spinal cord is part of the central nervous system and is found down the center of most of the vertebrae.

The spinal cord is made of an outer white matter region. This region is composed of mylineated axons.

The inner region is composed of grey matter. This region is composed of neuron cell bodies and dendrites.

In the center of the spinal cord is the central canal, where cerebrospinal fluid moves.

SPINAL CORD

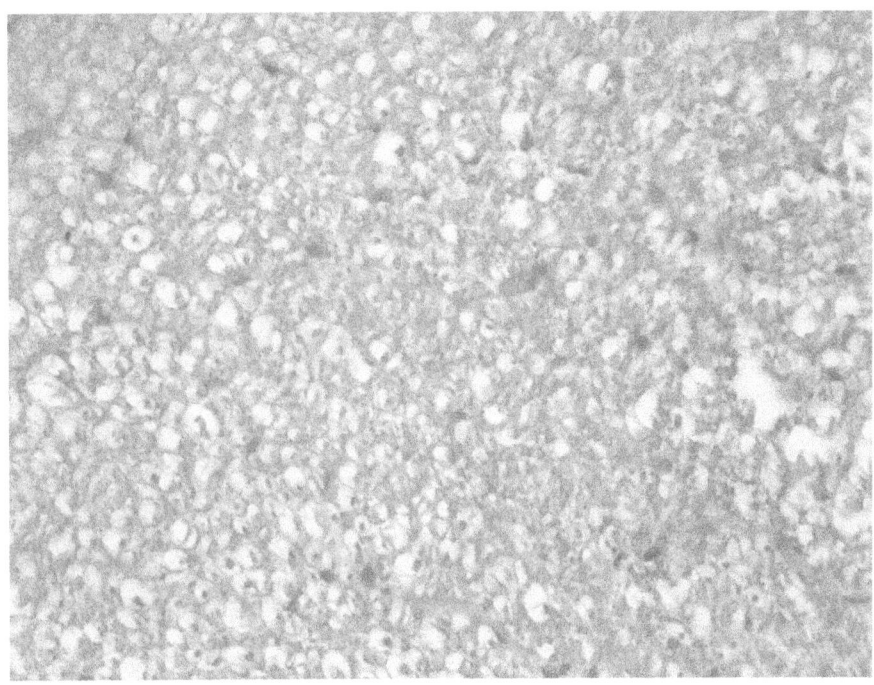

Spinal cord (white matter) at 400X

Many mylineated axons are shown in this slide

The spinal cord is part of the central nervous system and is found down the center of most of the vertebrae.

The spinal cord is made of an outer white matter region. This region is composed of mylineated axons.

The inner region is composed of grey matter. This region is composed of neuron cell bodies and dendrites.

In the center of the spinal cord is the central canal, where cerebrospinal fluid moves.

SPINAL NERVE

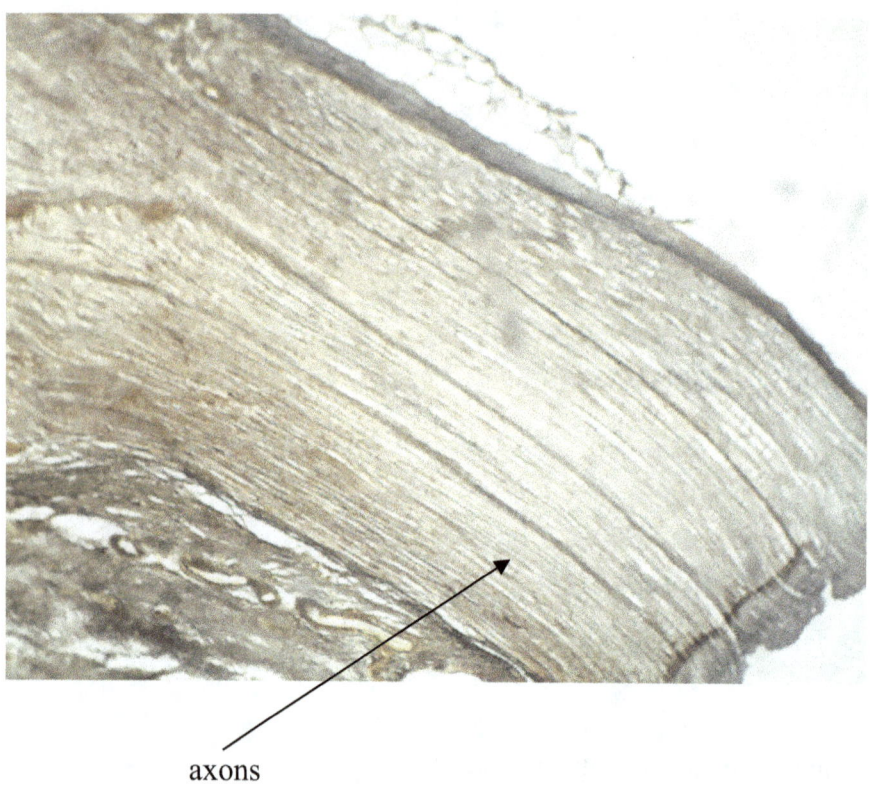

axons

Spinal nerve at 100X

Many axons can be seen running from left to right.

A spinal nerve is one of the nerves found in pairs down the spinal cord. Like other nerves it is composed of axons and myelin.

SPINAL NERVE

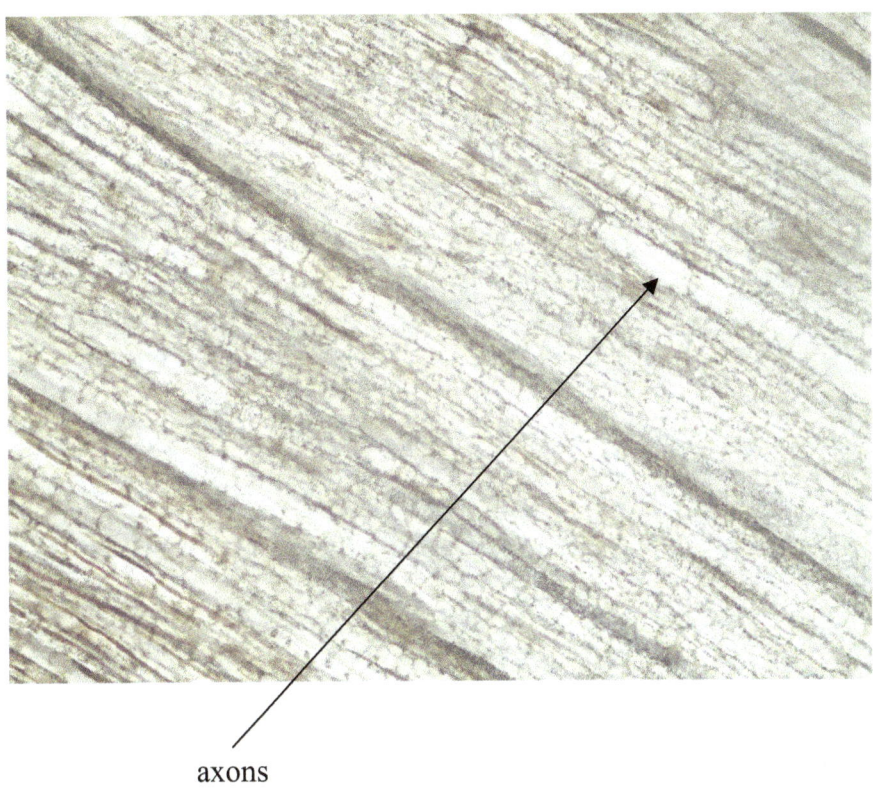

axons

Spinal nerve at 400X

A spinal nerve is one of the nerves found in pairs down the spinal cord. Like other nerves it is composed of axons and myelin.

SPLEEN

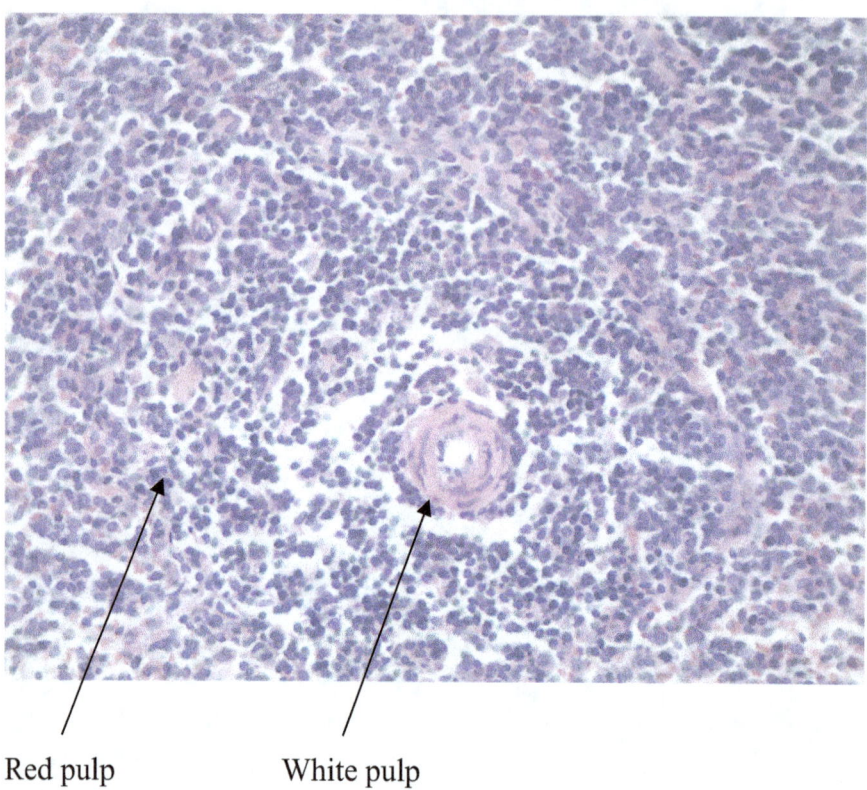

Red pulp   White pulp

Spleen at 400X

The spleen is located high in the upper left quadrant of the abdomen. Inside the spleen it is composed of white pulp areas full of white blood cells and red pulp areas made mostly of red blood cells. The white pulp surrounds the arterial blood supply.
The spleen will filter and remove materials not needed in the blood.

SPLEEN

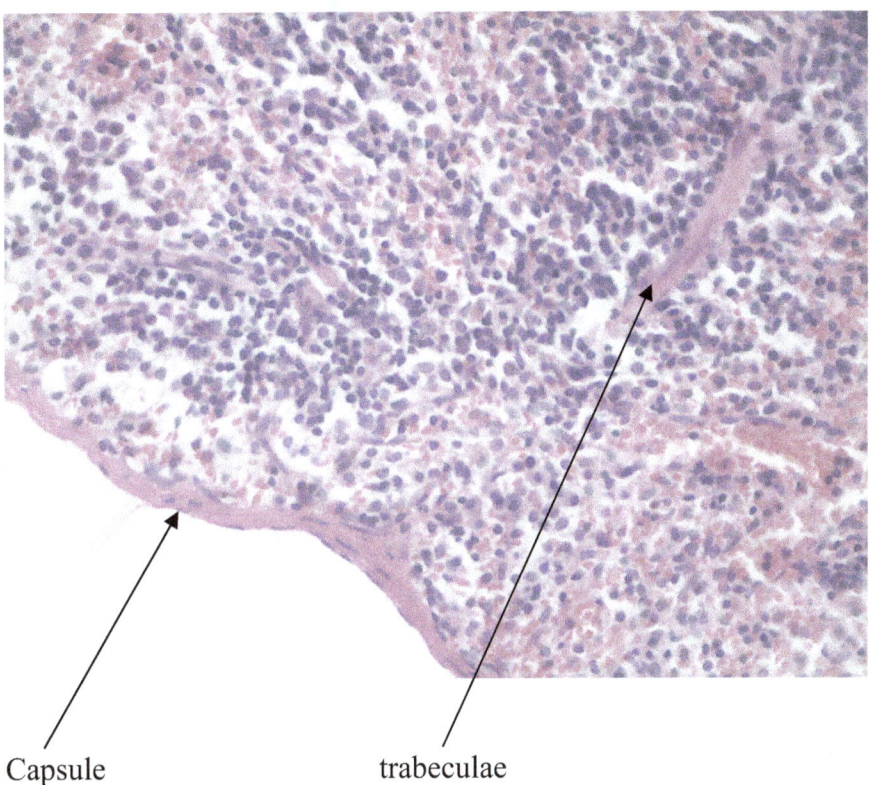

Capsule   trabeculae

Spleen at 400X

The spleen is located high in the upper left quadrant of the abdomen. Inside the spleen it is composed of white pulp areas full of white blood cells and red pulp areas made mostly of red blood cells. The white pulp surrounds the arterial blood supply.
The spleen will filter and remove materials not needed in the blood.

The capsule is an outer connective tissue layer surrounding the spleen.

SPONGY BONE

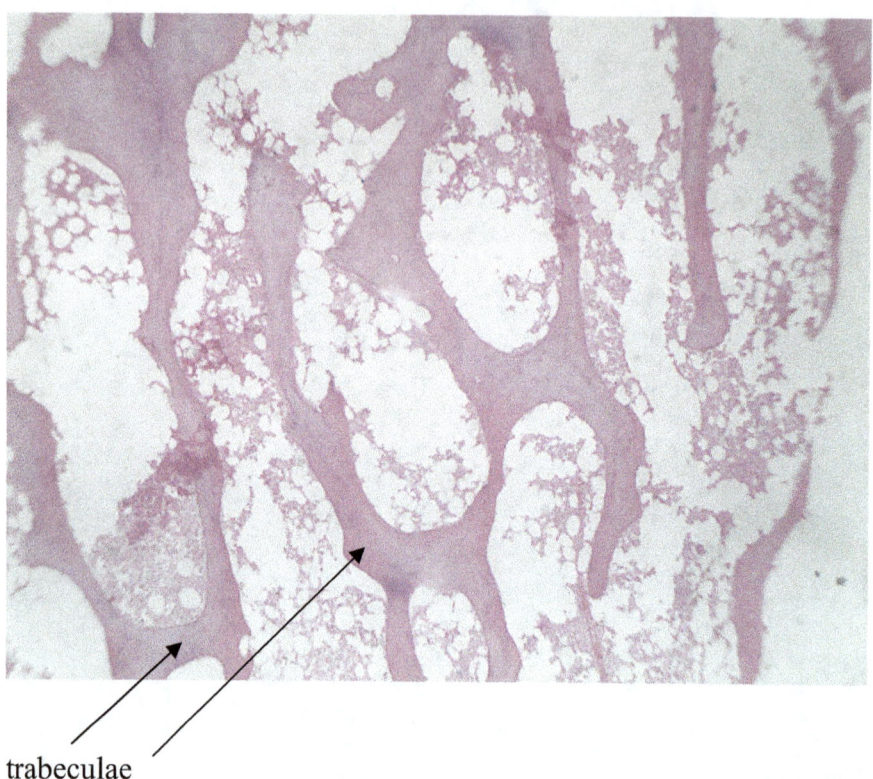

trabeculae

Spongy bone at 100X

Spongy bone is also called cancellous bone. This type of bone is composed of structures called trabeculae. Trabeculae are hard bony structures, which give strength to the bone.
It is called spongy bone because of its appearance, not because it is soft. This bone is not soft, but hard.

STOMACH

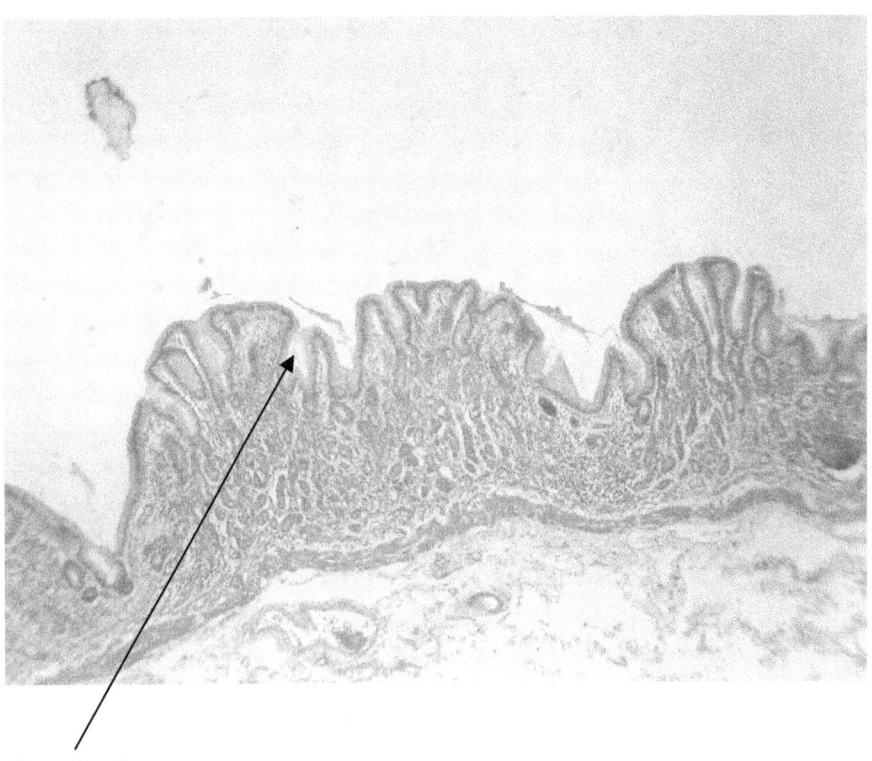

Gastric pits

Stomach at 40X

The stomach is a wide part of the GI tract and is a big mixing chamber. Little chemical digestion occurs in the stomach. The superior part of the stomach is called the fundus and the inferior (also distal) part is the pyloric region. The stomach contains folds to the inside called rugae (wrinkles). The inner lining of the stomach contains a large amount of mucous to protect it against acids and enzymes. Along this inner lining are many gastric glands and cells.

STOMACH

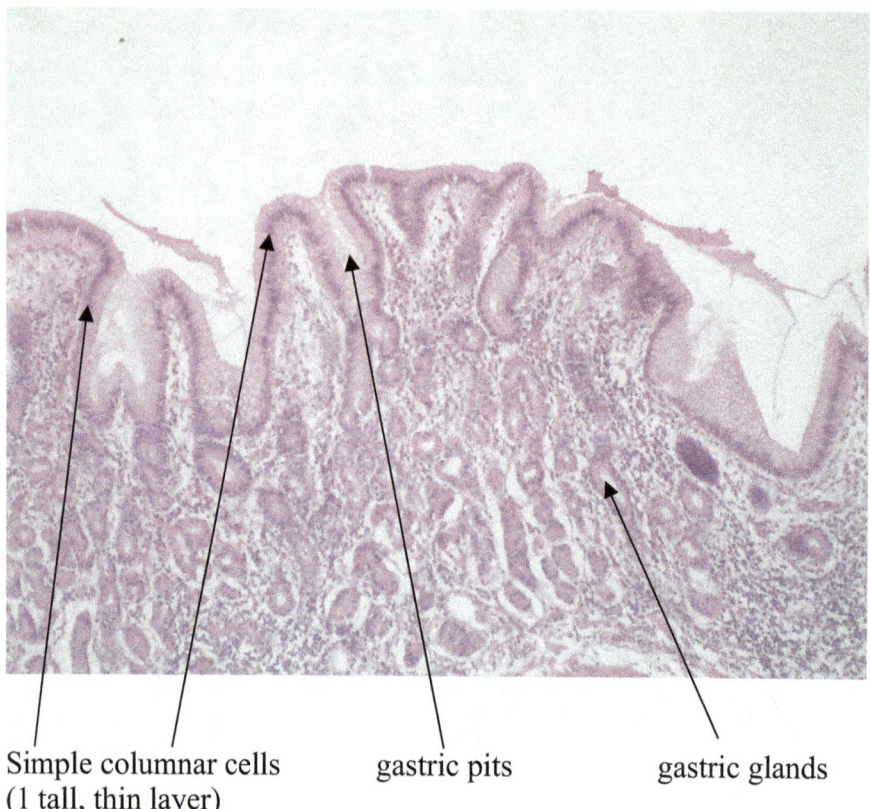

Simple columnar cells   gastric pits   gastric glands
(1 tall, thin layer)

Stomach at 100X

The stomach is a wide part of the GI tract and is a big mixing chamber. Little chemical digestion occurs in the stomach. The superior part of the stomach is called the fundus and the inferior (also distal) part is the pyloric region. The stomach contains folds to the inside called rugae (wrinkles). The inner lining of the stomach contains a large amount of mucous to protect it against acids and enzymes. Along this inner lining are many gastric glands and cells.

STOMACH

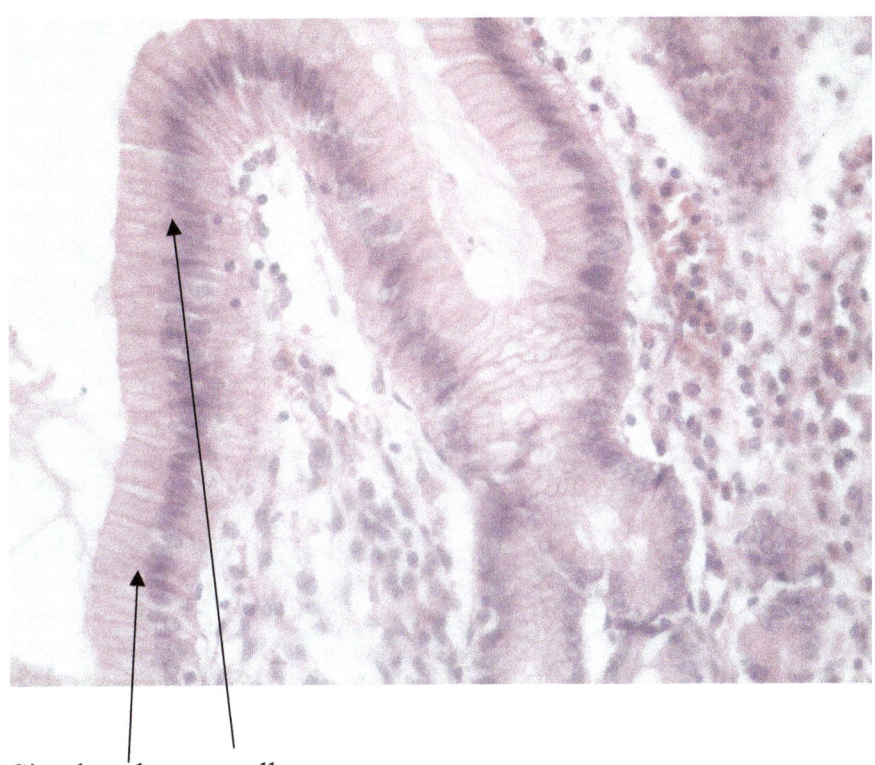

Simple columnar cells
(1 tall, thin cell layer)

Stomach at 400X

The stomach is a wide part of the GI tract and is a big mixing chamber. Little chemical digestion occurs in the stomach. The superior part of the stomach is called the fundus and the inferior (also distal) part is the pyloric region. The stomach contains folds to the inside called rugae (wrinkles). The inner lining of the stomach contains a large amount of mucous to protect it against acids and enzymes. Along this inner lining are many gastric glands and cells.

STOMACH

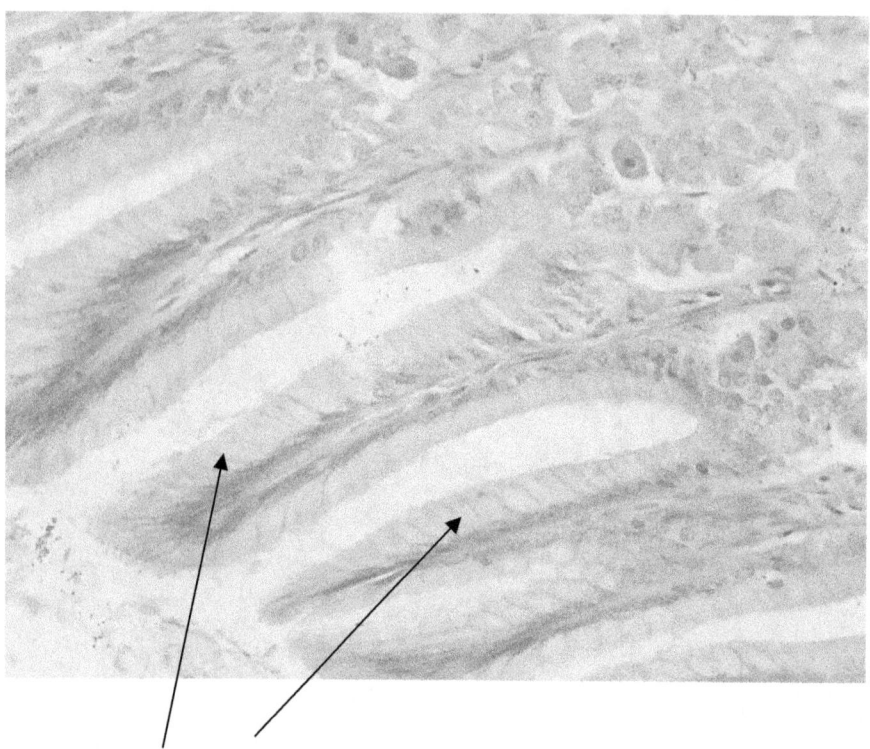

Simple columnar layer
(1 tall, thin cell layer)

stomach at 400X

The stomach is a wide part of the GI tract and is a big mixing chamber. Little chemical digestion occurs in the stomach. The superior part of the stomach is called the fundus and the inferior (also distal) part is the pyloric region. The stomach contains folds to the inside called rugae (wrinkles). The inner lining of the stomach contains a large amount of mucous to protect it against acids and enzymes. Along this inner lining are many gastric glands and cells.

STOMACH (fundus)

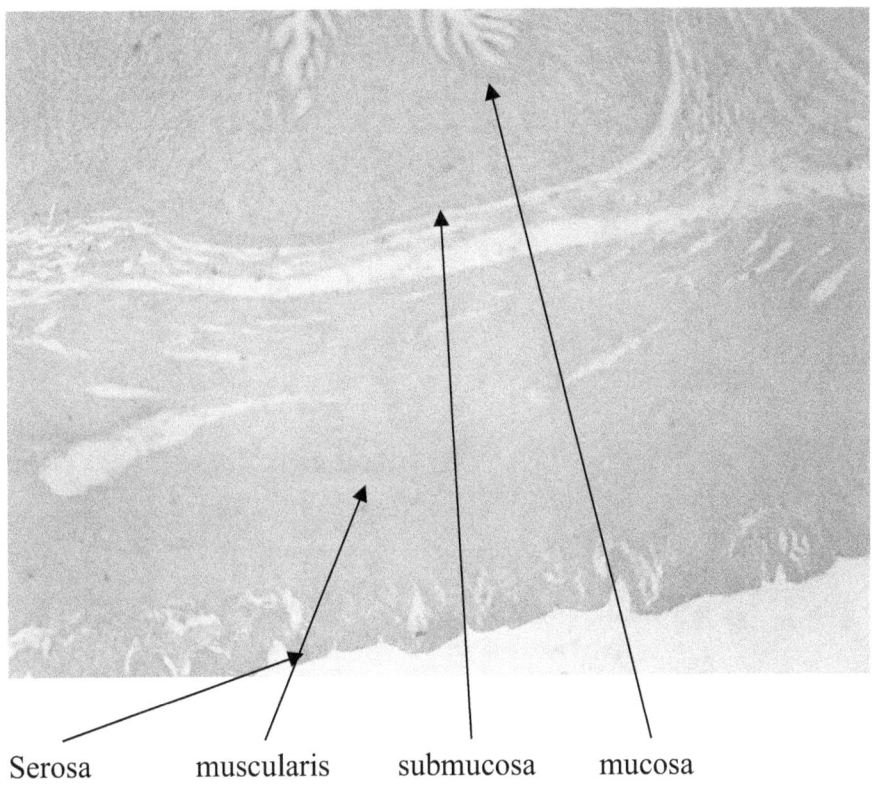

Serosa muscularis submucosa mucosa

Stomach (fundus) at 40X

The stomach is a wide part of the GI tract and is a big mixing chamber. Little chemical digestion occurs in the stomach. The superior part of the stomach is called the fundus and the inferior (also distal) part is the pyloric region. The stomach contains folds to the inside called rugae (wrinkles). The inner lining of the stomach contains a large amount of mucous to protect it against acids and enzymes. Along this inner lining are many gastric glands and cells.

SUBMANDIBULAR GLANDS

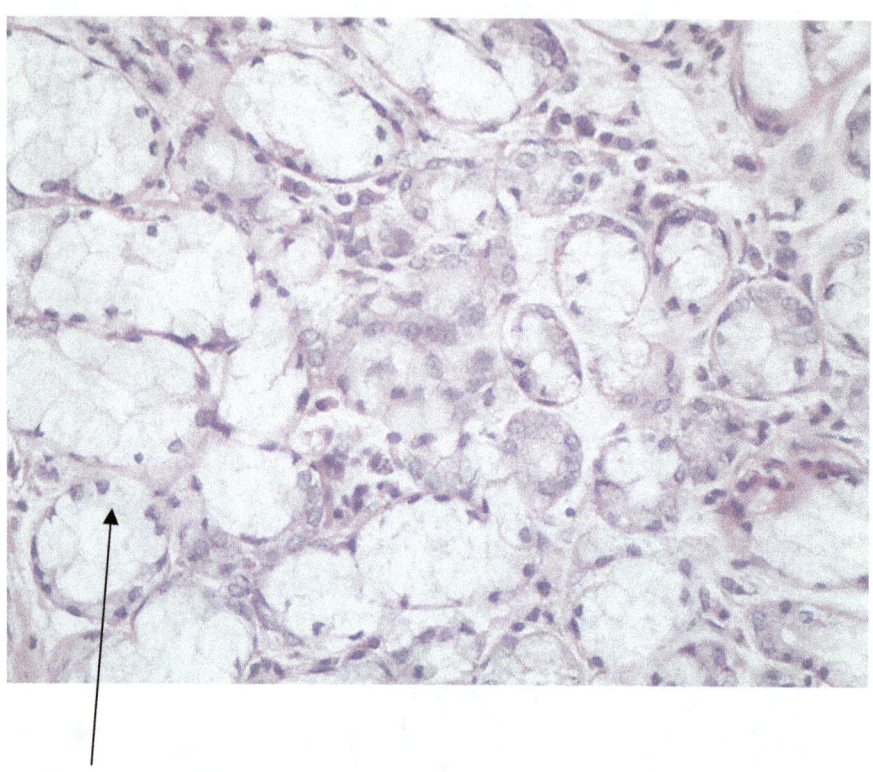

Simple cuboidal cells
(1 cube shaped layer)

Submandibular glands at 400X

The submandibular glands are just one of three sets of salivary glands. Along with the submandibular, we also have sets of sublingual and parotid salivary glands. These glands are always producing a watery secretion we call saliva. Saliva is mostly water, but it also possesses a small amount of digestive enzymes.

SWEAT GLANDS

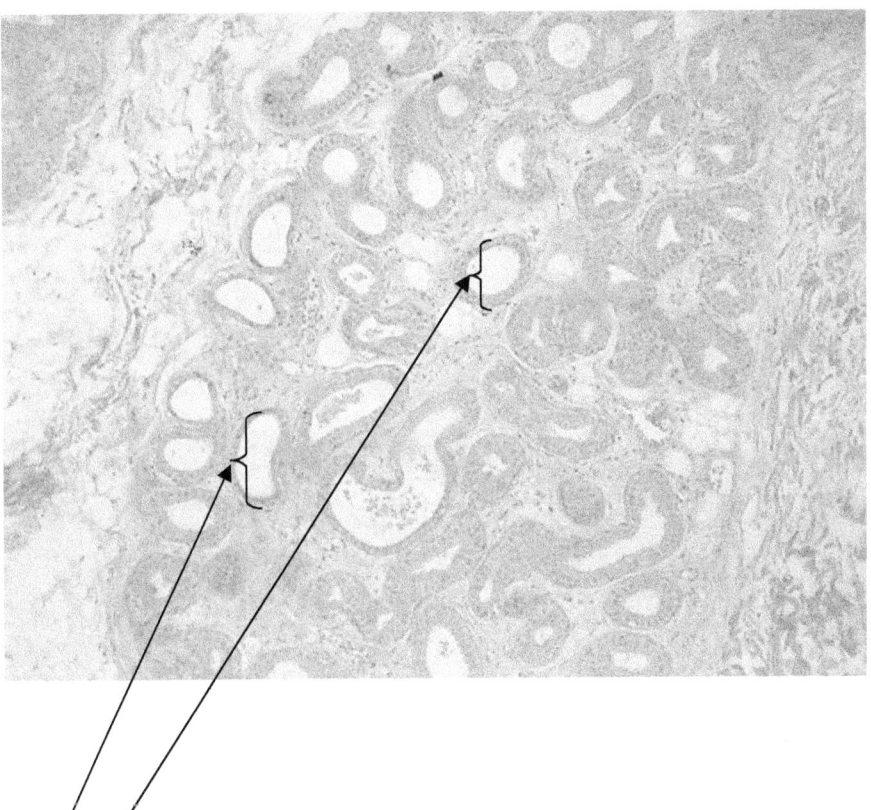

Sweat glands at 100X

Sweat glands are responsible for cooling the body. As these glands release water and other materials, the water will evaporate, and this will take heat with it.

SWEAT GLANDS

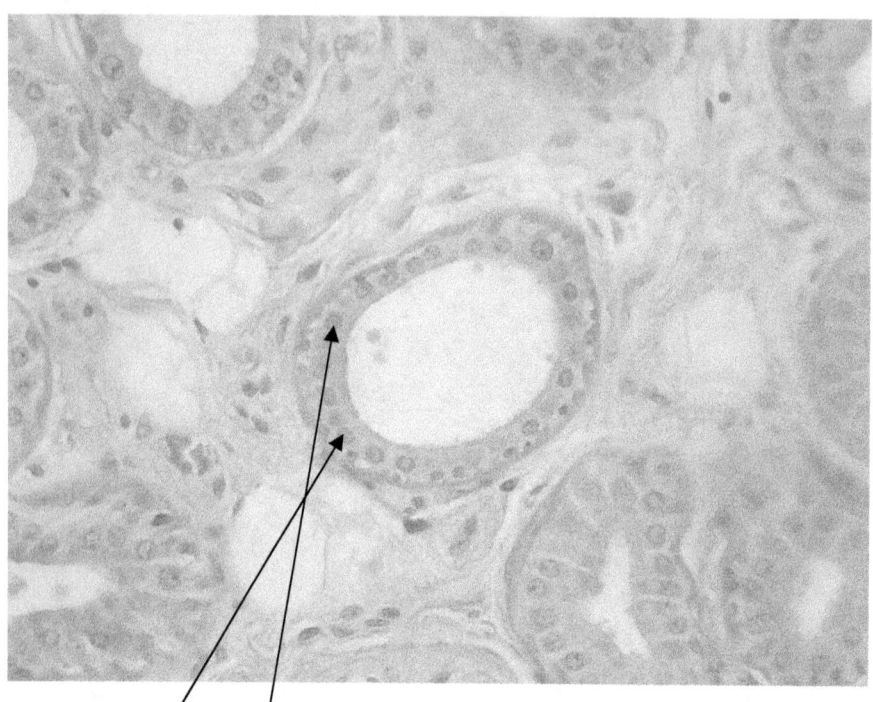

Simple cuboidal cells
(1 cube layer)

Sweat glands at 400X

Sweat glands are responsible for cooling the body. As these glands release water and other materials, the water will evaporate, and this will take heat with it.

TENDON

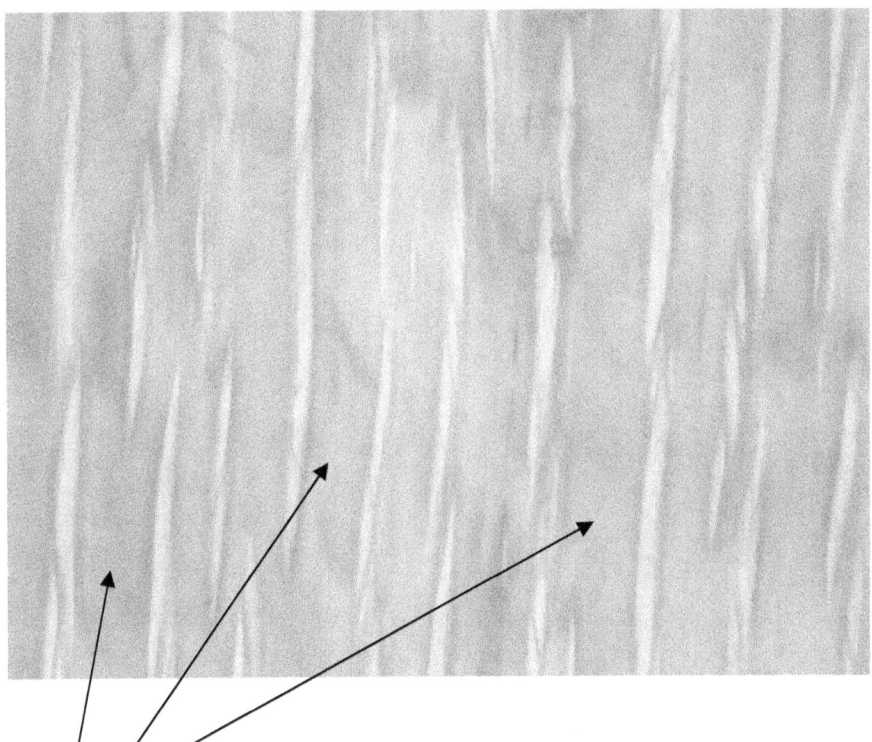

Collagen fibers

Tendon at 400X

A tendon is a dense, regular collagen arrangement. This means that many collagen fibers are tightly packed and arranged in the same direction. Notice how all of the collagen fibers run from the top to the bottom of the picture.

TESTIS

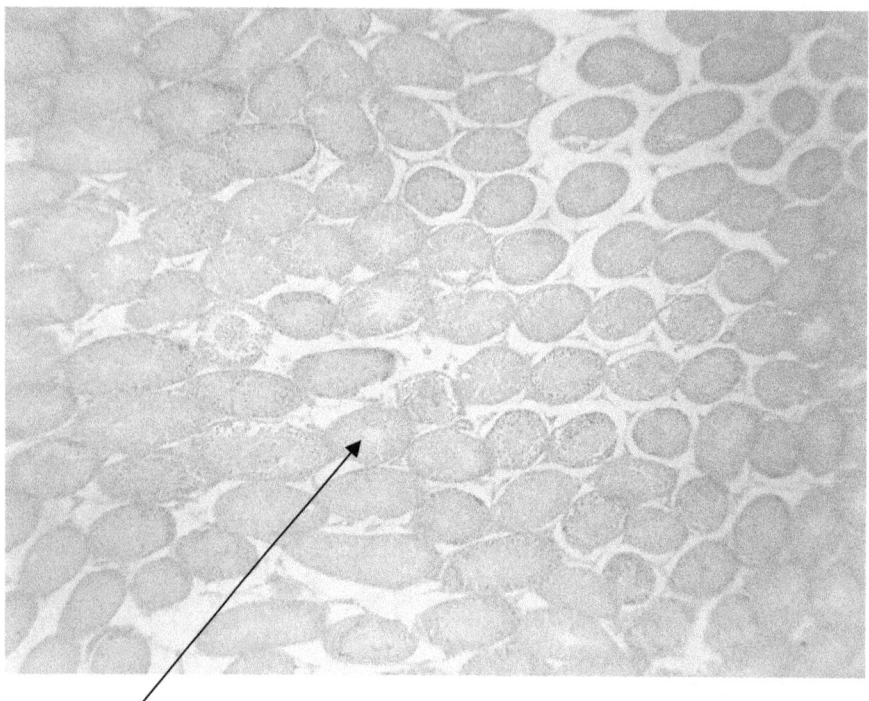

Seminiferous tubules

Testis at 40X

The testis are the paired gonads of the male reproductive system. The gonads are the organs responsible for producing the gametes (reproductive cells of the body). The testis are located outside of the male inside of a muscular sac called the scrotum. The testis are filled with seminiferous tubules and these tubes are where sperm cells are produced. Sperm cells only develop properly at 35 degrees Celsius (95 F) and this is why they are outside of the body. If the testis were inside the abdominopelvic cavity, they would be too warm, and the sperm cells wouldn't develop properly. Failure of the testes to descend is called cryptorchidism.

TESTIS

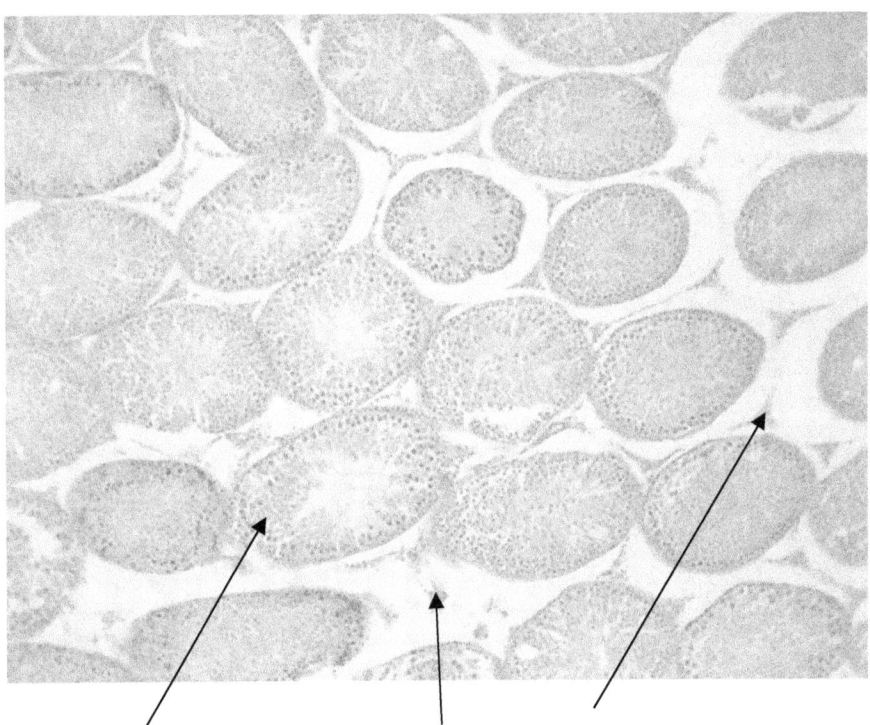

Seminiferous tubules   interstitial (Leydig cells)

Testis at 100X

The testis are the paired gonads of the male reproductive system. The gonads are the organs responsible for producing the gametes (reproductive cells of the body). The testis are located outside of the male inside of a muscular sac called the scrotum. The testis are filled with seminiferous tubules and these tubes are where sperm cells are produced. Sperm cells only develop properly at 35 degrees Celsius (95 F) and this is why they are outside of the body. If the testis were inside the abdominopelvic cavity, they would be too warm, and the sperm cells wouldn't develop properly. Failure of the testes to descend is called cryptorchidism. Leydig cells produce testosterone.

TESTIS

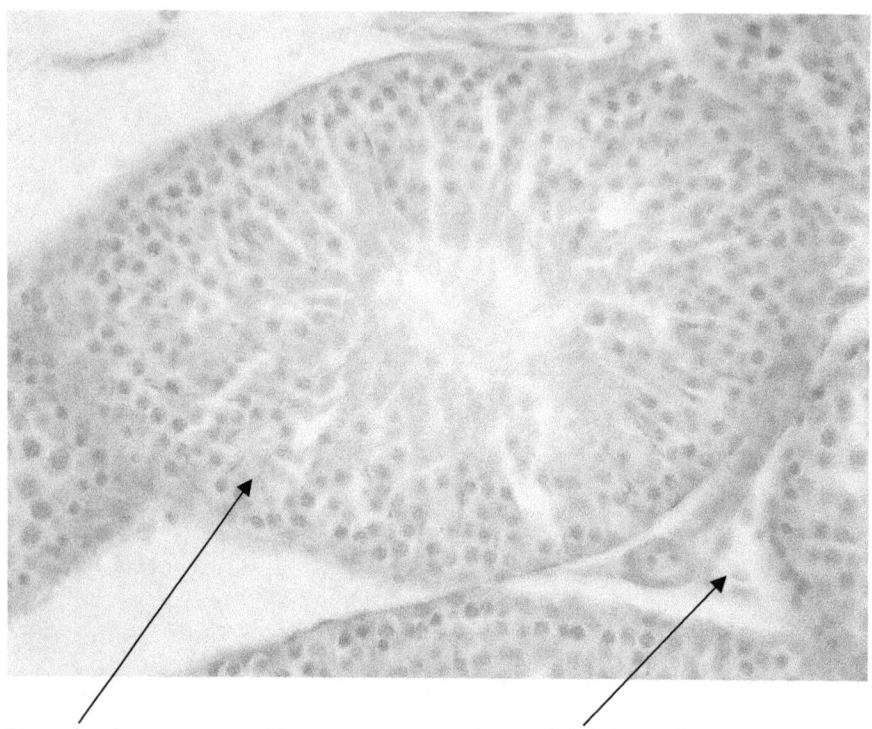

Developing sperm cells   interstitial (Leydig cells)

Testis at 400X

The testis are the paired gonads of the male reproductive system. The gonads are the organs responsible for producing the gametes (reproductive cells of the body). The testis are located outside of the male inside of a muscular sac called the scrotum. The testis are filled with seminiferous tubules and these tubes are where sperms cells are produced. Sperm cells only develop properly at 35 degrees Celsius (95 F) and this is why they are outside of the body. If the testis were inside the abdominopelvic cavity, they would be too warm, and the sperm cells wouldn't develop properly. Failure of the testes to descend is called cryptorchidism.

TESTIS

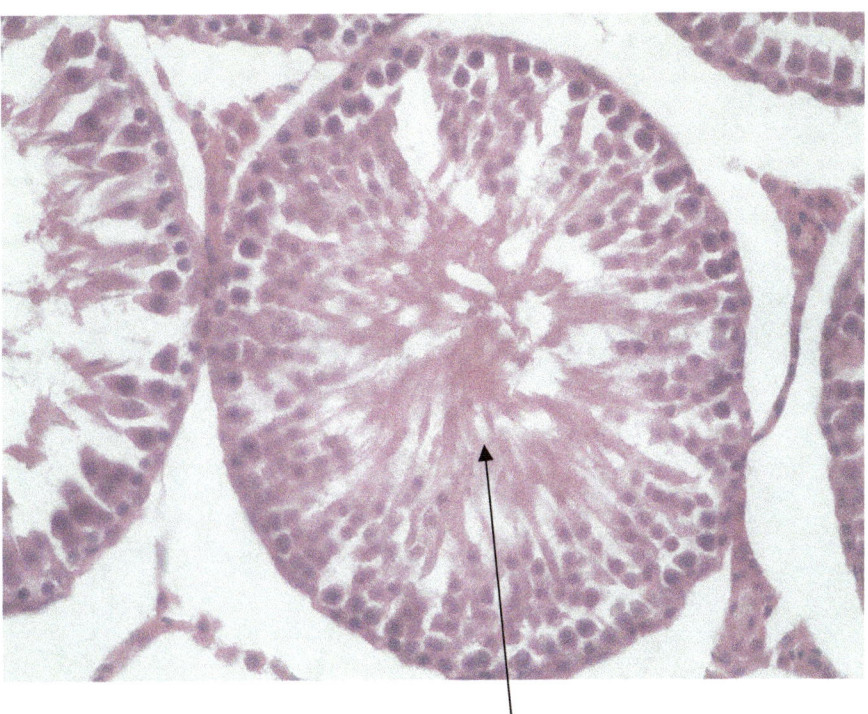

Testis at 400X   developing sperm cells

The testis are the paired gonads of the male reproductive system. The gonads are the organs responsible for producing the gametes (reproductive cells of the body). The testis are located outside of the male inside of a muscular sac called the scrotum. The testis are filled with seminiferous tubules and these tubes are where sperms cells are produced. Sperm cells only develop properly at 35 degrees Celsius (95 F) and this is why they are outside of the body. If the testis were inside the abdominopelvic cavity, they would be too warm, and the sperm cells wouldn't develop properly. Failure of the testes to descend is called cryptorchidism.

THREADS

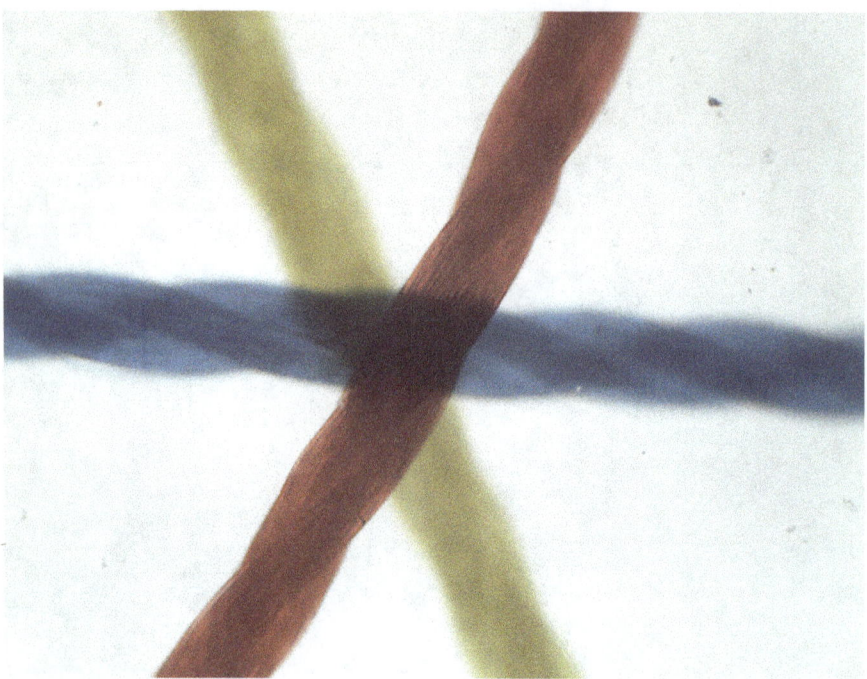

Threads at 40X

3 stacked threads are shown. Notice how when one is in focus the others aren't.

THYMUS GLAND

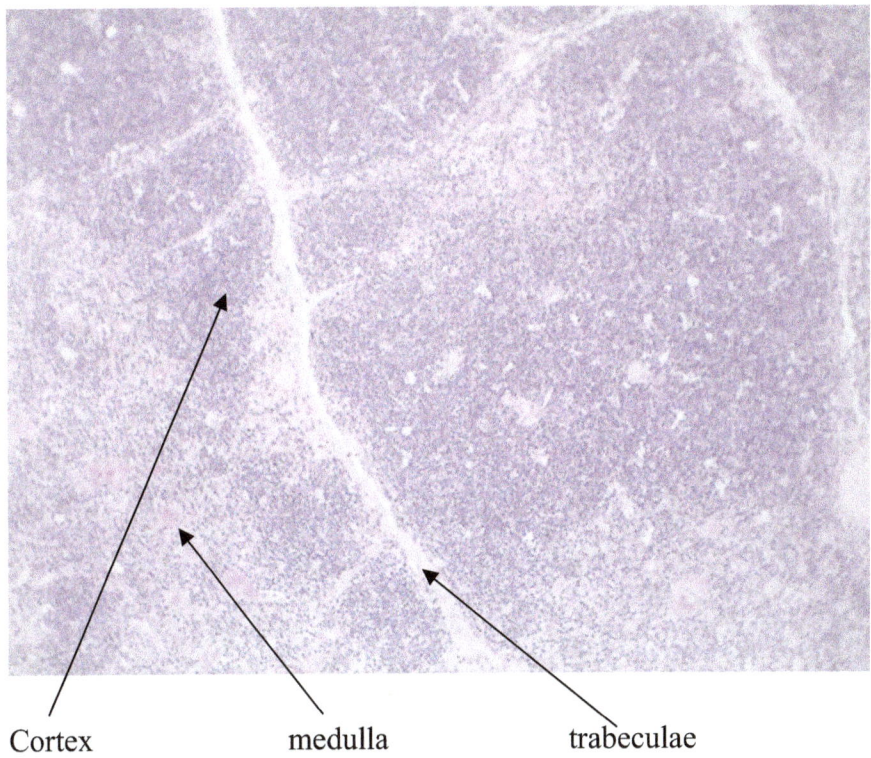

Cortex   medulla   trabeculae

Thymus gland at 40X

The thymus gland is a very important part of the lymphatic system. This gland is where T cells mature.

The hormone thymosin is produced here.

THYMUS GLAND

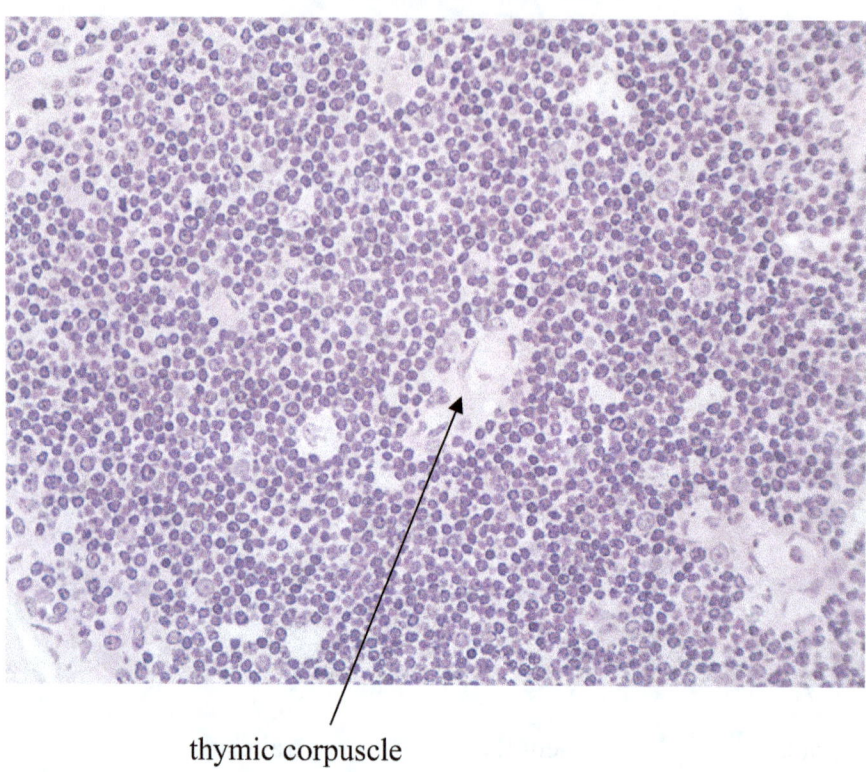

thymic corpuscle

Thymus gland at 400X

The thymus gland is located just superior and anterior to the heart. It is larger when we are young and decreases in size as we get older.

THYMUS GLAND

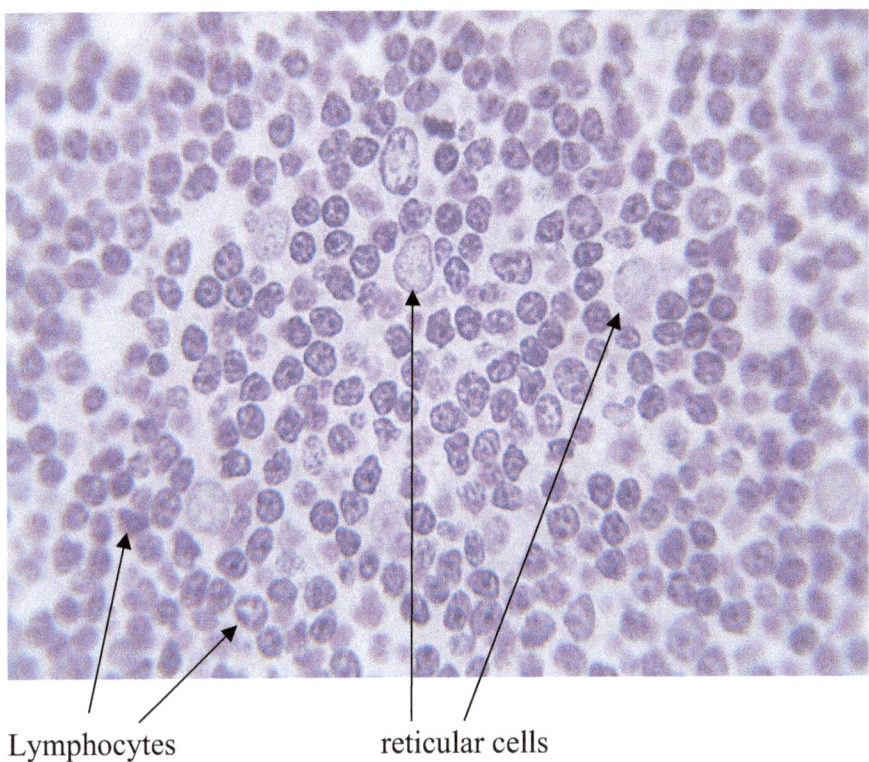

Lymphocytes   reticular cells

Thymus gland at 1000X

THYROID GLAND

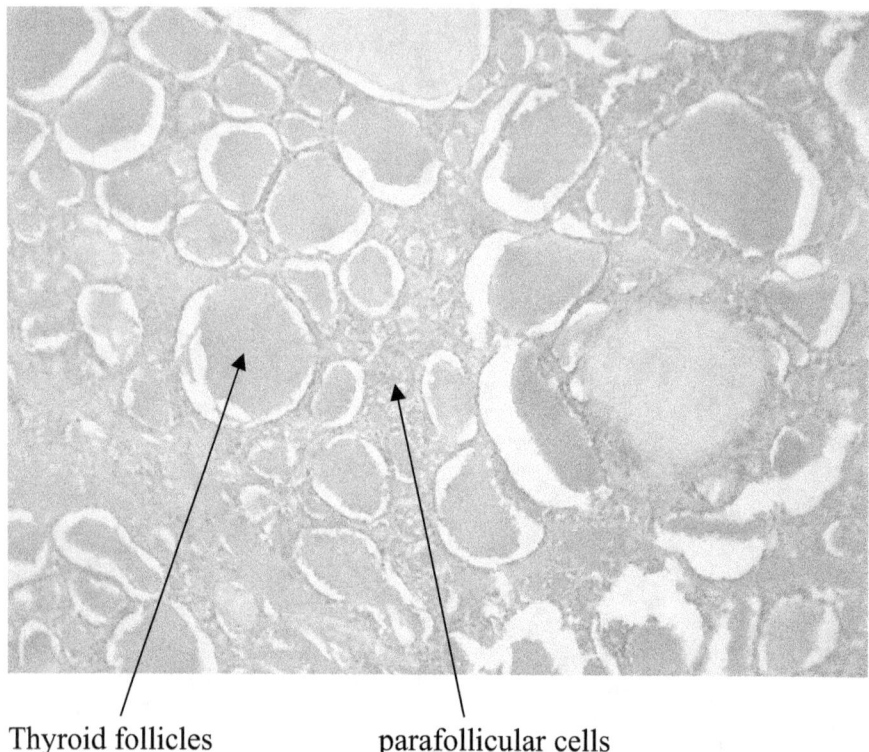

Thyroid follicles   parafollicular cells

Thyroid gland at 100X

The thyroid gland is responsible for producing thyroid hormone and calcitonin. Thyroid hormone is also called T3 (triiodothyronine) and T4 (tetraiodothyronine). These hormones are responsible for regulating metabolism. These hormones regulate how many mitochondria cells we have and how active they are. When we are young these hormone levels are higher. We need these hormones to be higher at a young age, because they are needed for growth to occur properly.

THYROID GLAND

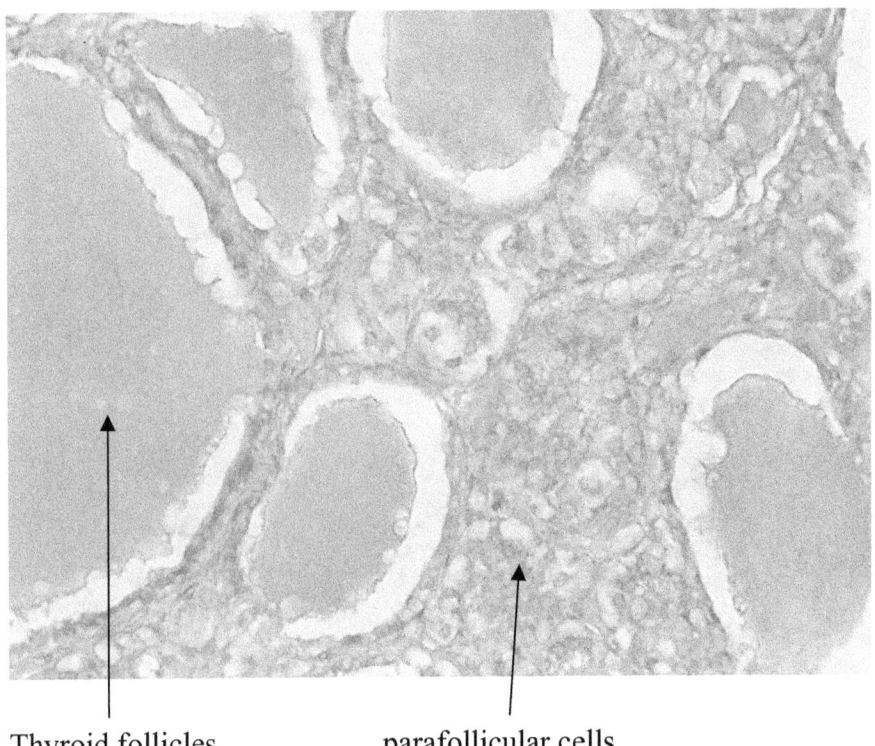

Thyroid follicles   parafollicular cells

Thyroid gland at 400X

The thyroid gland is responsible for producing thyroid hormone and calcitonin. Thyroid hormone is also called T3 (triiodothyronine) and T4 (tetraiodothyronine). These hormones are responsible for regulating metabolism. These hormones regulate how many mitochondria cells we have and how active they are. When we are young these hormone levels are higher. We need these hormones to be higher at a young age, because they are needed for growth to occur properly.

TONGUE (taste buds)

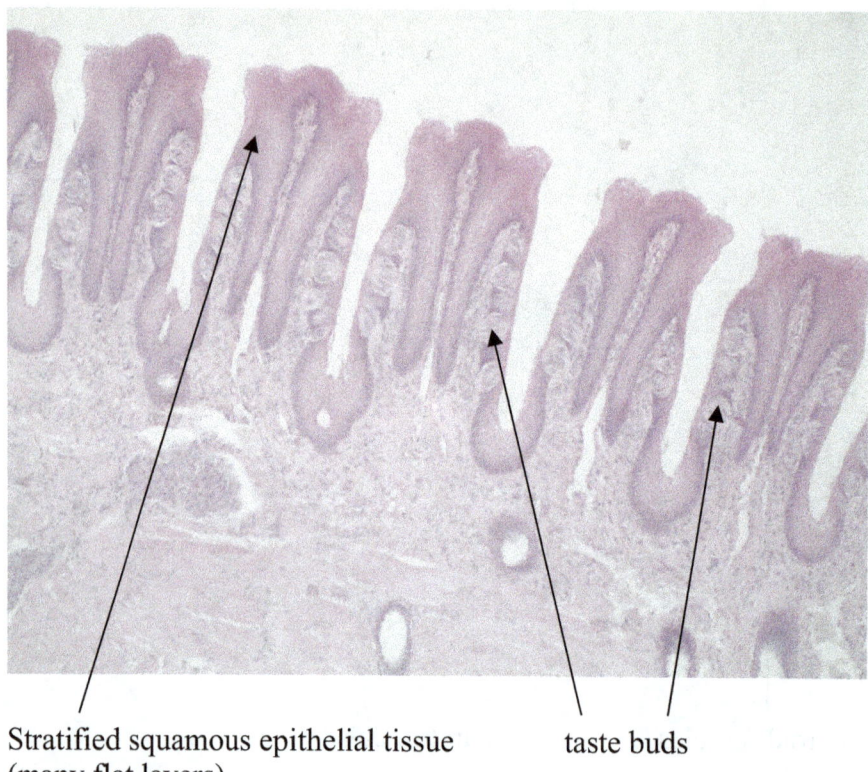

Stratified squamous epithelial tissue (many flat layers)

taste buds

Tongue (taste buds) at 100X

The tongue is covered with a stratified squamous epithelial tissue. This thick layer is needed to protect the tongue against abrasion and other forms of damage.

TONGUE (taste buds)

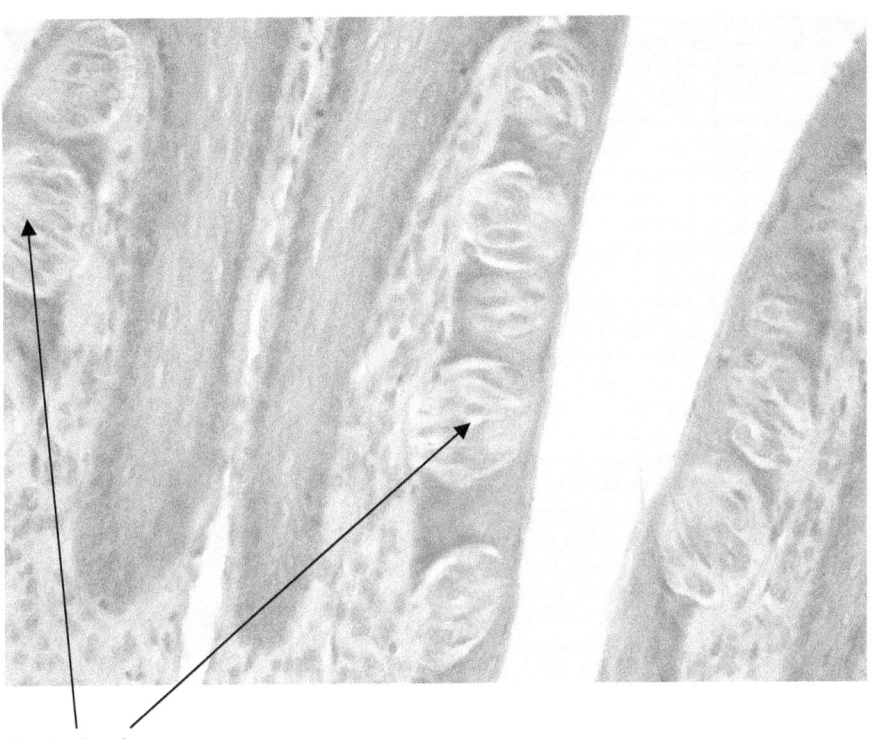

Taste buds

Tongue (taste buds) at 400X

The tongue is covered with structures called papillae. These papillae come in four different shapes: filiform, fungiform, vallate and foliate. The taste buds are found along the lateral margins between the papillae. The taste buds are located on the lateral margins, so they are protected from damage. Taste buds are the sensory structures responsible for taste.

TONSILS

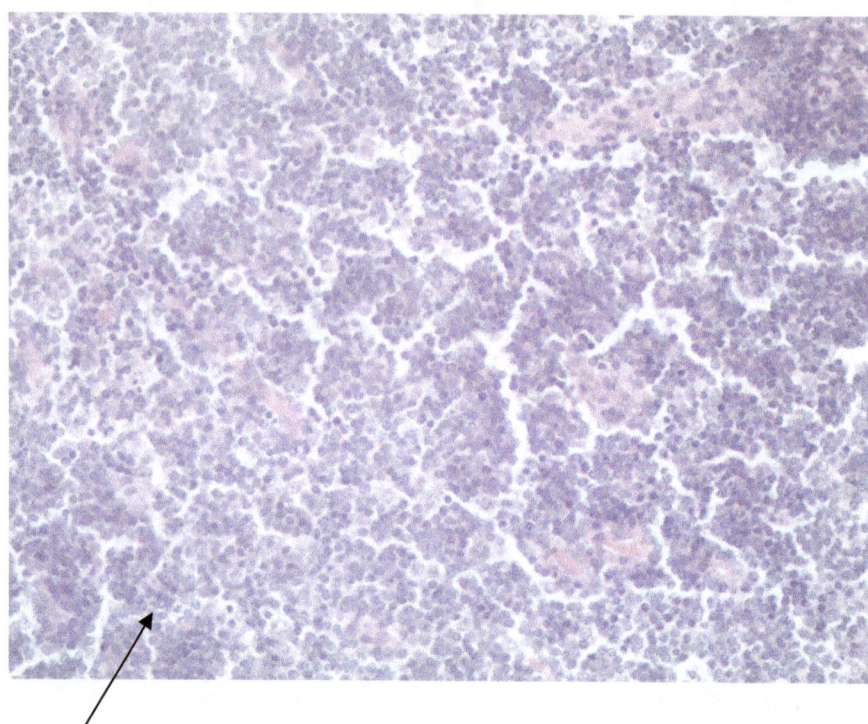

lymphocytes

Tonsils at 400X

The human body contains three sets of tonsils. Some are found in the oral cavity and some in the pharynx (throat). The different tonsils are pharyngeal (adenoids), lingual and palatine (tonsils).

The pharyngeal are located in the pharynx and sometimes cause problems with breathing. The lingual are located on the tongue and the palatine are the ones seen to the rear of the oral cavity.

The tonsils are large collections of white blood cells beneath a thin mucous membrane. As foreign invaders try to enter the body through the digestive and respiratory system, these white blood cells will catch and destroy them.

TONSILS

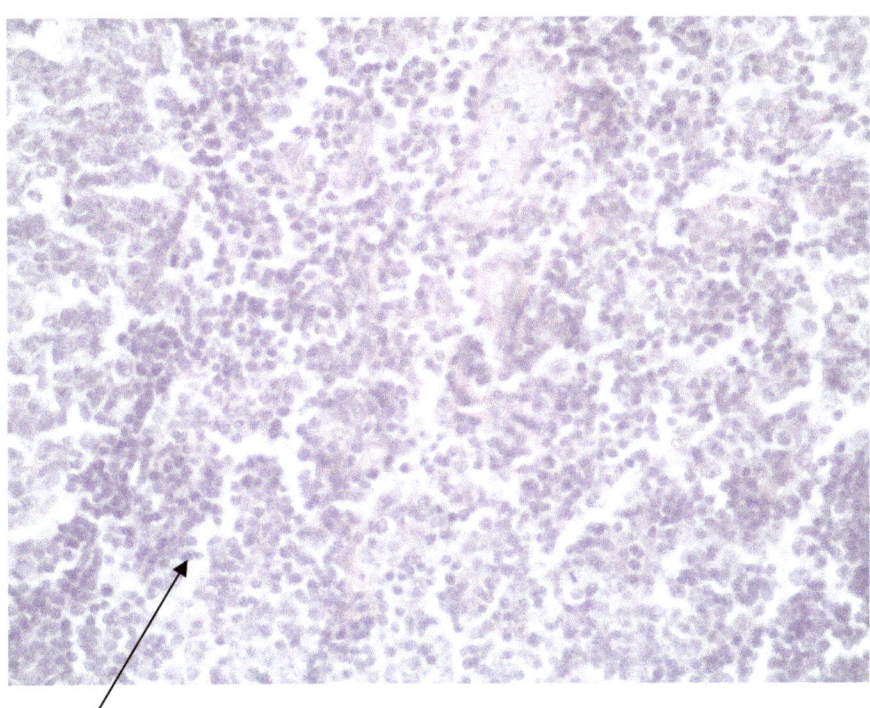

lymphocytes

Tonsils at 400X

The human body contains three sets of tonsils. Some are found in the oral cavity and some in the pharynx (throat). The different tonsils are pharyngeal (adenoids), lingual and palatine (tonsils).

The pharyngeal are located in the pharynx and sometimes cause problems with breathing. The lingual are located on the tongue and the palatine are the ones seen to the rear of the oral cavity.

The tonsils are large collections of white blood cells beneath a thin mucous membrane. As foreign invaders try to enter the body through the digestive and respiratory system, these white blood cells will catch and destroy them.

TRACHEA (cilia)

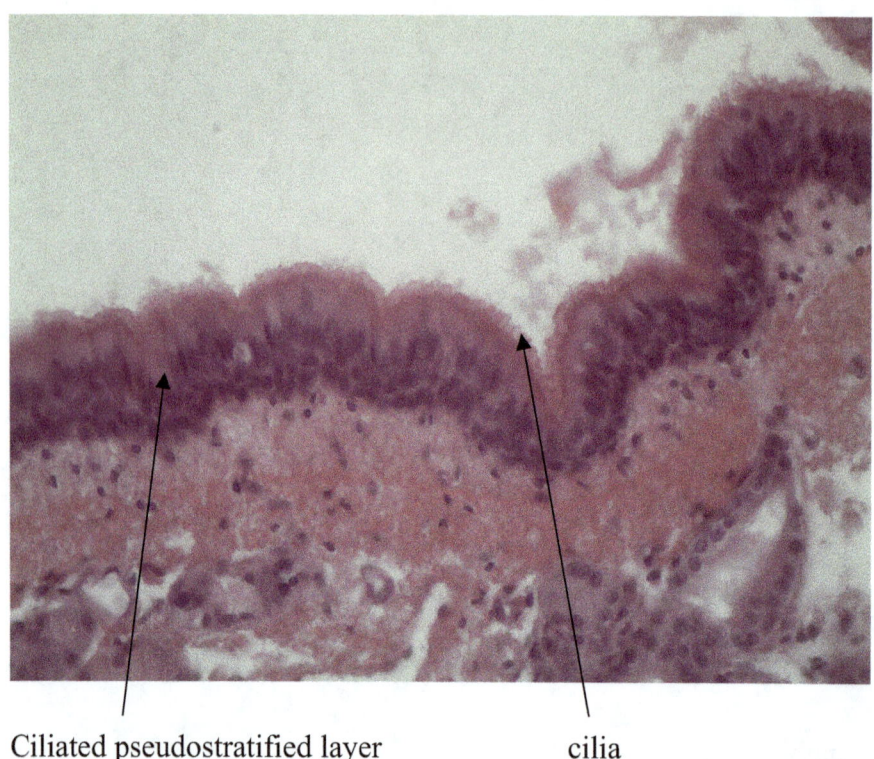

Ciliated pseudostratified layer   cilia
(1 cell layer)

Trachea (cilia) at 400X

The trachea is also called the windpipe. This air passageway is filled with mucous and cilia. As we breathe, the mucous will trap foreign particles suspended in the air. As the mucous cleans the air the cilia move the particles in a superior direction away from the lungs. This forms an escalator of mucous, always cleaning the upper air passageways.

URETER

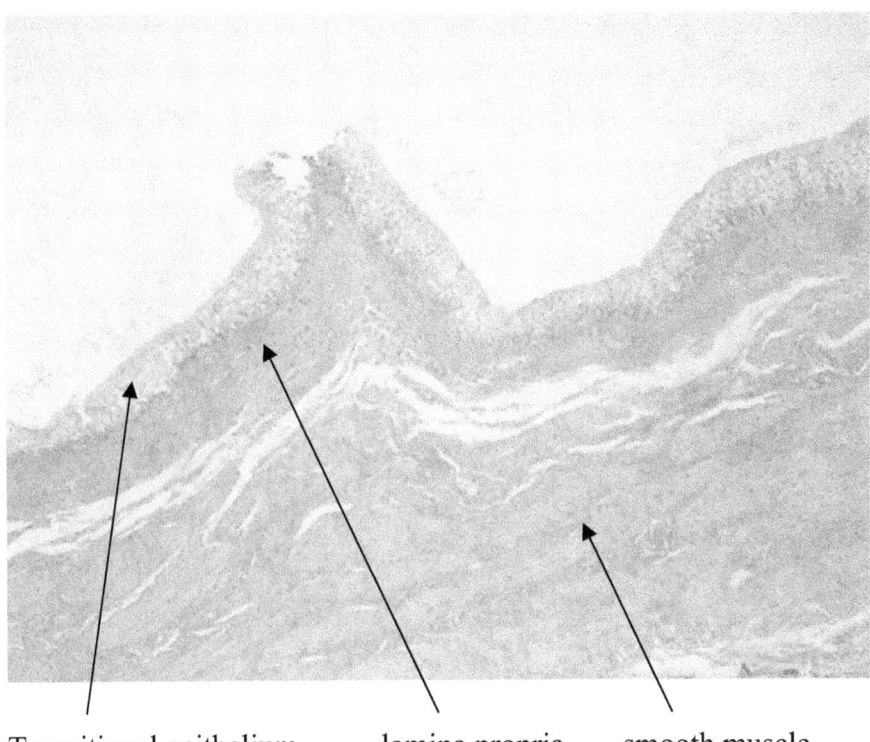

Transitional epithelium   lamina propria   smooth muscle

Ureter at 100X

The ureters are hollow muscular tubes connecting the kidneys and the urinary bladder. The smooth muscle of the ureters will push urine from the kidneys into the bladder.

URETER

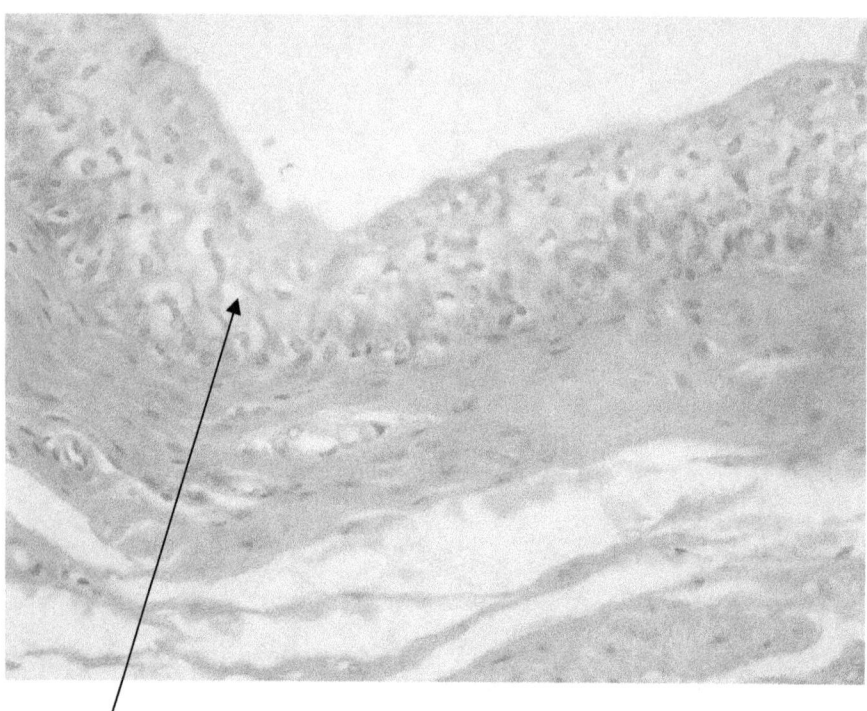

Transitional epithelium

Ureter at 400X

Transitional epithelium allows for expansion inside hollow organs. The number of epithelial cell layers is thick when a structure is empty, and the cells unfold and flatten as a structure fills.

VAGINA

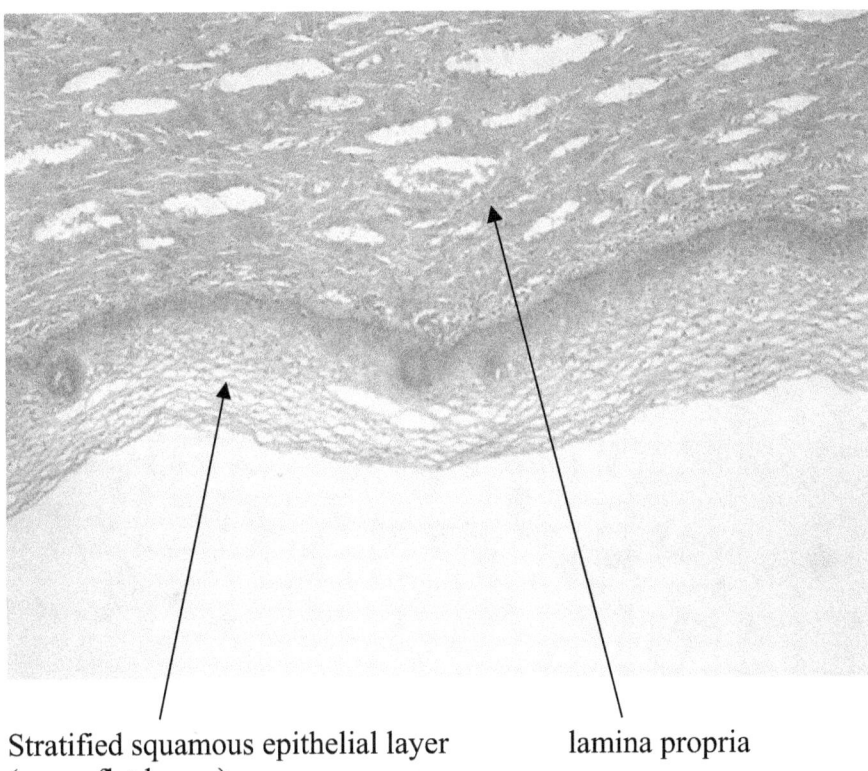

Stratified squamous epithelial layer (many flat layers)　　lamina propria

Vagina at 100X

The inner layer of the vagina is stratified squamous to protect from abrasion. Many cell layers are much better than one or only a few, when it comes to protecting deeper structures.

VAGINA

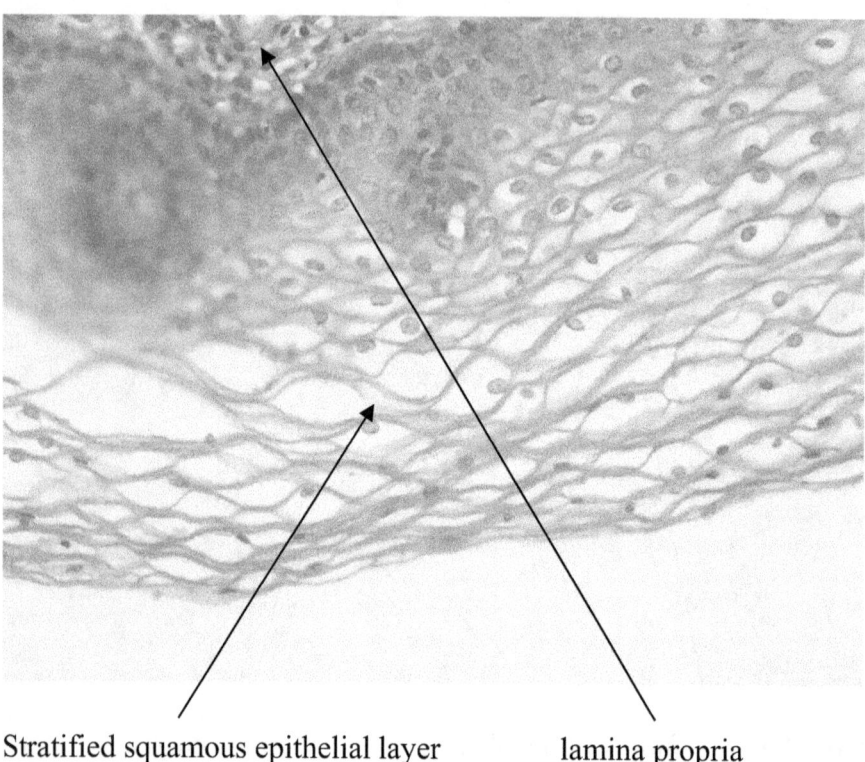

Stratified squamous epithelial layer (many flat layers)   lamina propria

Vagina at 400X

Notice how the deeper cells are cuboidal but the superficial ones are squamous. Always look at the superficial layers, when determining cell shape.

VENA CAVA

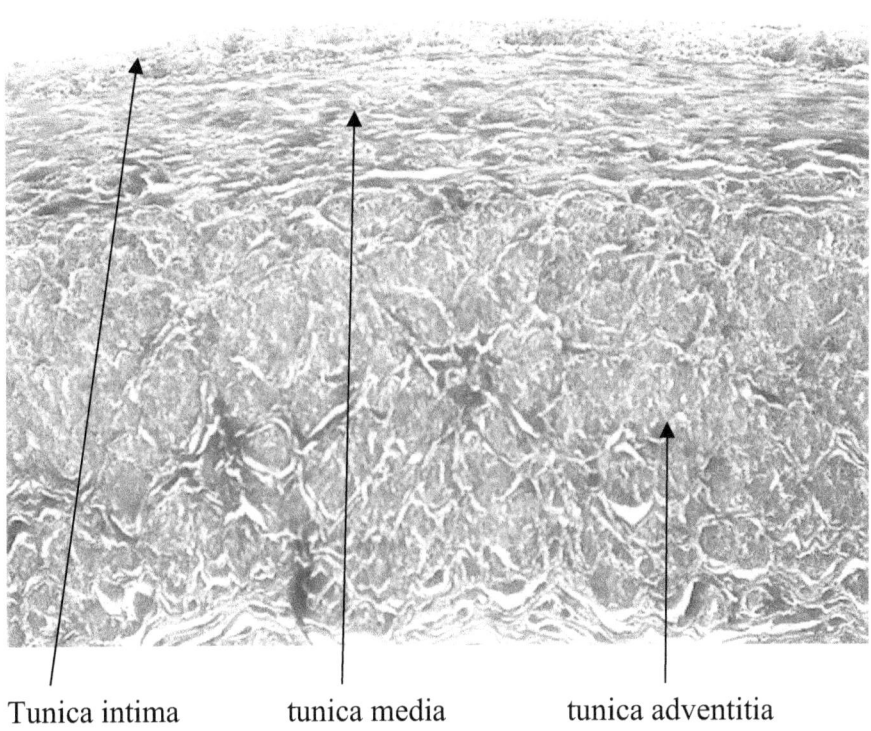

Tunica intima   tunica media   tunica adventitia

Vena cava at 400X

The vena cava are large veins which return blood back to the right atrium of the heart.

www.ingramcontent.com/pod-product-compliance
Lightning Source LLC
Chambersburg PA
CBHW051539240526
45465CB00028B/1085